AF357307

Mad About CRACKERS

Simple recipes for healthy raw snacks the whole family will love based on FRUITS, VEGETABLES and SEEDS

First self-published 2022

Photos by Margo.

The book design, cover & art was co-created by Margo (author), Solaja Slobodan (graphic designer), Sanjida Smrity (graphic designer) and Edita.artdiary (digital artist).

A catalog record for this book is available from Slovak National Library (www.snk.sk)

ISBN: 978-80-570-3758-3

Content

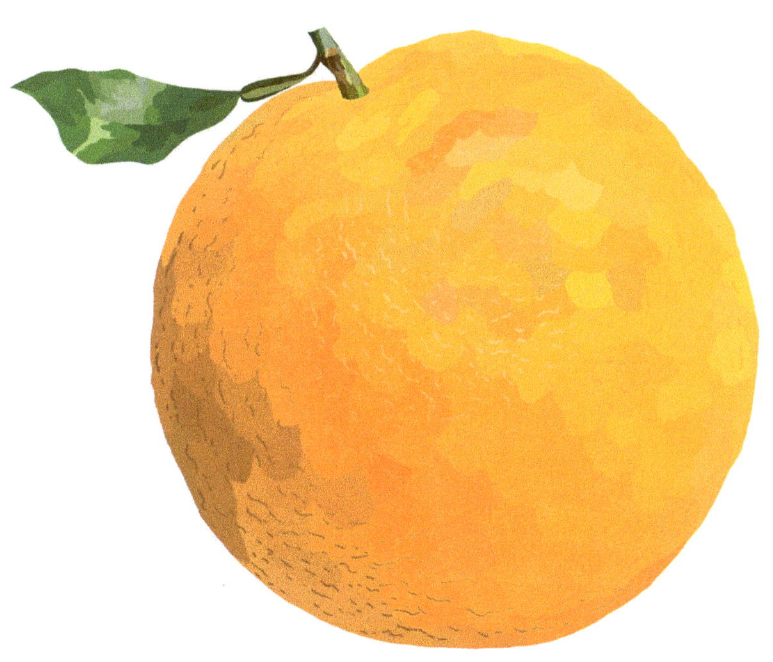

5

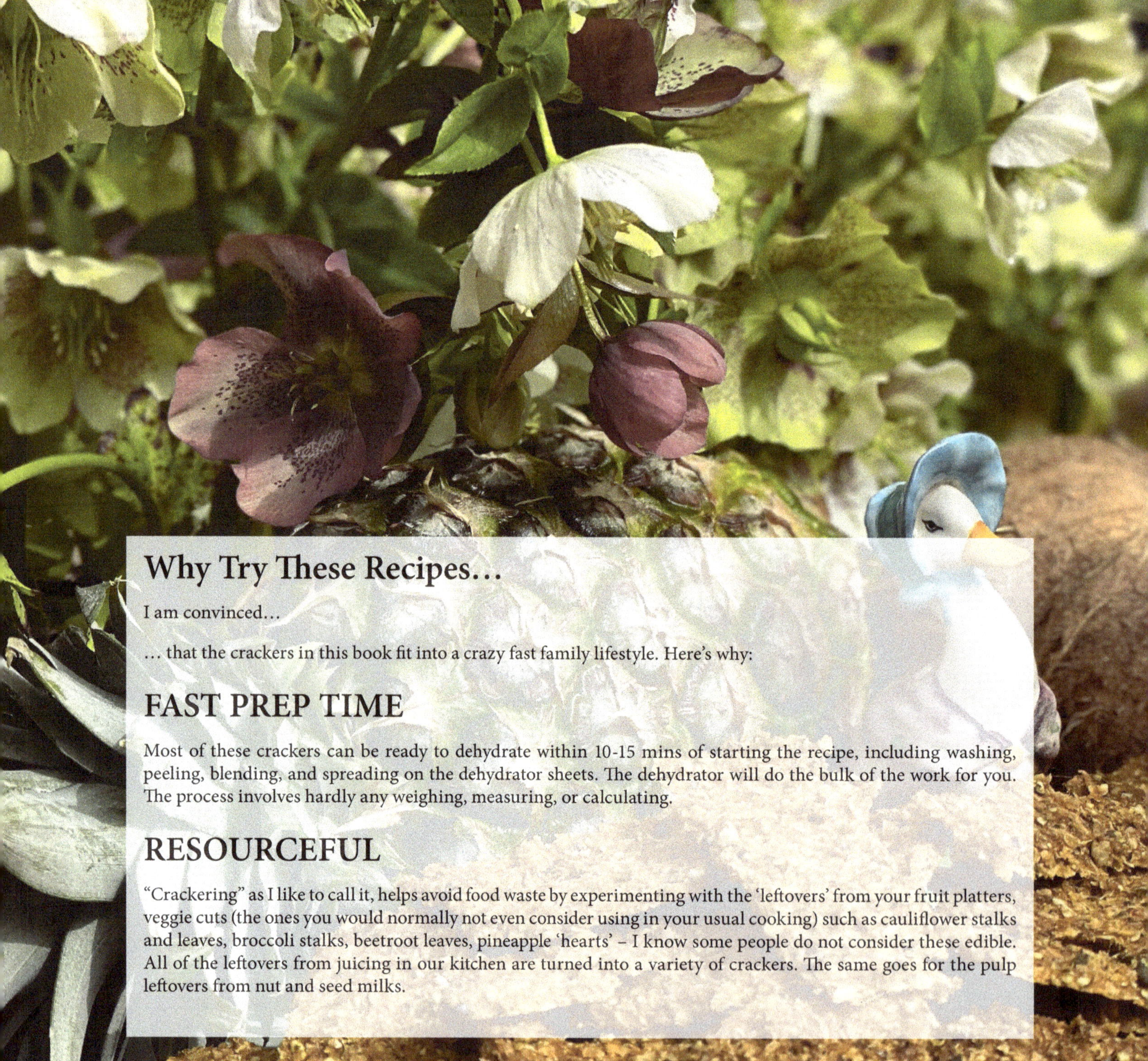

Why Try These Recipes…

I am convinced…

… that the crackers in this book fit into a crazy fast family lifestyle. Here's why:

FAST PREP TIME

Most of these crackers can be ready to dehydrate within 10-15 mins of starting the recipe, including washing, peeling, blending, and spreading on the dehydrator sheets. The dehydrator will do the bulk of the work for you. The process involves hardly any weighing, measuring, or calculating.

RESOURCEFUL

"Crackering" as I like to call it, helps avoid food waste by experimenting with the 'leftovers' from your fruit platters, veggie cuts (the ones you would normally not even consider using in your usual cooking) such as cauliflower stalks and leaves, broccoli stalks, beetroot leaves, pineapple 'hearts' – I know some people do not consider these edible. All of the leftovers from juicing in our kitchen are turned into a variety of crackers. The same goes for the pulp leftovers from nut and seed milks.

If your garden gives you an abundant harvest… so much that no way can it all get eaten in its fresh state… and if there is only so much space in your freezer…

I would say it's time to make crackers!

LONG-LASTING

Of course, the shelf life is limited by hungry snackers, but if very well dehydrated and stored properly, dehydrated goodies last weeks or even months.

VERSATILE

The versatility of these crackers is endless.

Try and test. For kids, I find thicker crackers are often liked more- as they do not break easily, creating hardly any crumbs. Some kids clearly prefer the chewier texture.

For a more gourmet 'grown-up' experience – thin delicate crispy crackers are a nice variation. (Yep, you also end up consuming less even though you're enjoying them for longer.) You can make sticks, squares, rectangles, triangles, even circles (any shape at all if you dry them to a softer consistency and then cut shapes out with scissors or use your favorite cookie cutter), then continue drying to final crispiness. Tiny, medium, big, long, funky…

As you will see in one of the fruity recipes – one can dehydrate fruit to a certain chewy texture and then create funky rolls, which may remind kids of commercially sold fruity roll-ups.

Crackers are a filling and balanced snack. They can be used as deserts, party food, lunch box fillers, trail plate additions, emergnecy food or healthy and light 'travel' (on the go) snacks.

One can even create an ultra-runner's snack by adding extra calorie-dense ingredients and maybe some protein powders into the basic cracker recipe.

TASTY

Follow the recipes in this book and discover that crackers convert fruit and veg into fun, tasty treats for even fussy eaters and veg-phobics. If your child likes strawberries, raspberries – or any fruit really – they will never know their favorite cracker also contains lots of parsnips, carrots, spinach, pumpkin, etc.

SUPERHEALTHY

Made with fresh vegetables, fruits, seeds, herbs and spices, these crackers are just a mass of vitamins, minerals, micronutrients, fiber, and healthy fats.

Zero additives, preservatives, colorings, nasty 'E' numbers or the hidden sugars, oils, or excessive salt you may find when looking more closely at labels on the snacks on the supermaket shelves.

5-a-day has never been so easy!

… because raw fruits and veggie crackers will be something your kids will keep asking for. I am convinced we are onto a simple solution to the question (or quest even!) you as a parent have been on for a while… The 5-a-day quest.

When I see "5-a-day" printed on the packaging of processed foods it makes me smile and wonder! (And let's be honest, it is not a rare finding because from a marketing point of view, such a line has the power to tip the shopper's scale in favor of the product.)

But what does 5-a-day really mean? What does it mean to you?

"5-a-day" is the title of national campaigns in countries such as the U.K., USA, Germany, France to encourage consumption of at least five portions of fruits and vegetables each day. These were inspired by the WHO recommendation that individuals consume a minimum of 400 g of fruit and vegetables per day. And NO… potatoes in the form of fries do not count in case you were wondering… In Australia a similar campaign was initiated called "Go for 2&5" encouraging adults to consume at least two servings of fruit and five servings of vegetables each day. The size of portions differs from country to country in some of these campaigns… So what if we try to make it simple for ourselves?

Instead of counting portions, grams, calories, let's look at the overall content of our daily plates? What is the percentage or ratio of fresh fruits and vegetables compared to processed foods you and your kids consume? To begin with, I am daring to suggest aiming for at least half of your meals to be fresh fruits or vegetables. Does it sound like too much? (Maybe too little to some?) When I feed kids, toddlers, and babies, as a general rule I consider ONE portion to be approx. equal to the size of their fist. When it comes to food, children are still pure and unconditioned beings. Let's give them the chance to decide for themselves what they think of specific fruits and vegetables and how they taste to them! There are thousands of beautiful fruits out there in the world. As a parent or carer, please give them the opportunity to TRY and taste them! Why just five? Five or seven? It is just a guideline. More is better. Let's help the kids of the world develop a lifestyle where counting fruits and veggies is not needed. Fresh, clean, ripe fruits and vegetables will be the food of choice for them, natural to reach for, to be nourished and powered by. My cracker ideas and your creative efforts to make them may be a tool that will help along the way…

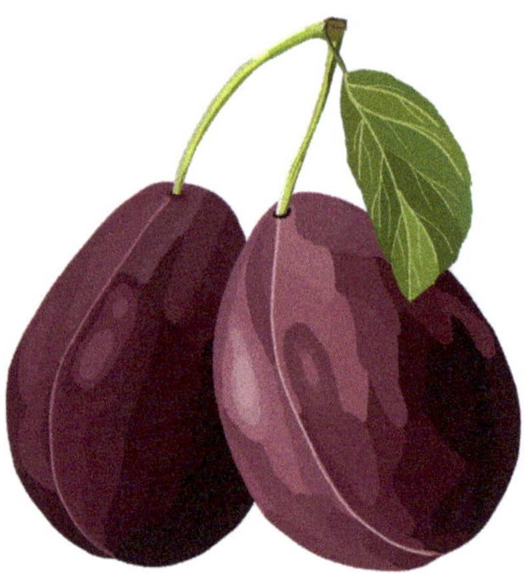

Let's CRACKER ON together to make the world a better place…

I wholeheartedly believe that a happy and healthy start in life with a clean and pure diet sets your child up for the future and will help you succeed in raising happy healthy kids. This is a subject so very close to my heart and I am passionate about spreading awareness and teaching young parents how to actually start to feed their little babies from day ONE. *(My first little book Go Wild is a simple weaning guidebook. It is a collection of my personal ideas and thoughts about baby foods. Go Wild explains in an uncomplicated way how to safely include fruits, vegetables, even raw leaves and flowers of edible 'wild' and garden plants, into the meals and diets of babies, toddlers, breastfeeding mothers and the whole family, with great healing benefits.)*

In the world today, words and phrases such as food intolerance, eczema, autoimmune disease, allergy, food allergen, food desensitization, child epilepsy are frequently used and sadly not so shocking anymore: which is why knowledge about safe foods is crucial.

And yes – I imagine that most parents know about the importance of their kids' nutritional needs. Yet it is easy to get overwhelmed when accessing information from various sources.

Reading food labels can be confusing.

A clean, balanced diet is key to healthy eating habits!

Early childhood is an important time to establish healthy eating patterns!

Eating behaviors and meal habits in early childhood have an impact on children's eating patterns and food preferences in adulthood.

We live in a busy world now. Parents have less and less time to prepare healthy homemade meals. I do not blame them! It can be a challenge to encourage children to eat vegetables and fruits every day if you're in a rush and have many other parenting and life challenges to attend to.

It is a good idea to offer children a variety of healthy foods such as fruits and vegetables which are easy to eat and require only simple washing or peeling. Maybe arrange them on a table in a visible place where it is easy for them to reach throughout the day, anytime when the child is hungry. This way parents can shape their children's food preferences since kids are more likely to enjoy those foods they are offered regularly. Healthy snacks make healthy happy kids.

Additionally, children learn eating habits through observation…

The whole process of making one batch of crackers – from the moment of washing the fruit and veg to placing the trays in the dehydrator – takes me 10-15 mins overall. Especially if good music is playing.

Of course, it can take longer if you share this activity with the little ones and turn the crackering into sweet, family-gathering fun – a hands-on project for your kids.

Let them have their say on which pieces of fruit and veg should go in the crackers. Let them witness the transformation of foods they know into something new and very yummy.

It encourages their creativity, curiosity and – as far as the bigger picture is concerned – one day they'll be interested about where food comes from, safe food production, gardening, and harvesting, etc.

And even bigger still… questions about world economies and planet ecology, once they've grown up a little more. These fresh, young open minds are our hope. It is our responsibility to shape them right.

I know, I know, I got carried away – I just like to foresee the future and visualize the possible positive outcome of seeds planted in young, pure, angelic minds.

We all hear this information and I think some of us 'sense' it on a deeper level too: the disconnect from nature is a real issue these days.

I consider myself lucky – being a gardener, fascinated by Nature from an early age, led by my parents to watch seeds grow into beautiful fruits that I get to harvest with my own hands.

I treasure this fascination.

I cultivate my own appreciation and gratitude for Mother Nature and her wonders, the self-healing capacity we all possess, as well as the incredible compatibility and connection of human beings to all plants and the rest of nature that surrounds us. Natural food is just part of this compelling wonder.

By the way – part of early healthy eating habits is to teach children to recognize hunger signals. Bribing or punishing kids to eat everything on their plate sends them the wrong message about how much they need to eat until they are full.

I think it is wise to allow kids to listen to their own hunger cues.

Part of the whole 'healthy kids for life' deal is active play and sports time. Please encourage them to leave the house and play in the garden, run around with friends, join athletic or dance teams… all these will help to reduce the risk of becoming overweight, plus this way kids also develop better social skills, self-confidence, and emotional stability which can lead to strong self-esteem.

Gardening can be wonderful outdoor fun.

Just this one particular point would definitely help make the world a better place. Just think about the clean air, free clean roads, seas, and skies that would result if the fruits and vegetables we eat didn't have to be imported from other continents to our table.

At the same time, all of us together will produce so much less packaging waste. We will help preserve cleaner air for our future generations once our snacks and their packaging are no longer produced in big factories and driven to supermarkets in big trucks or on airplanes from foreign countries. Is this thought appealing?

It is very exciting for me. Knowing that every little step and improvement matters. The compound positive effect of it all on this beautiful green planet – our home – can be massive.

Think of the ripple effect happening in a BIG WAY on many levels.

It can all start with a cracker.

My husband says I was "born to cracker!"

Years ago, long before we met, he was diagnosed with an autoimmune disease. When he nibbles on my crackers – the usual worry of him possibly having some strange, horrible allergic reaction to the hidden preservatives/colorants/additives in many branded snacks goes away. Like a heavy, dark and frightening cloud of constant worry for my loved one being lifted off my mind…

Do your kids suffer from allergies, eczema, etc? Making crackers for them, snacks they will love and seek is an easy win-win.

If I only inspire a couple of you to try and improve your and your kids' health and the future wellbeing of your body through healthier (and very yummy) snacking – my mission is complete!

We will plant more fruit trees and expand the lung capacity of Mother Earth. We will create beauty to look at. We will harvest not only beautiful fruits and vegetables every season, but experience JOY and SATISFACTION of good deeds well done. People who have a healthy relationship with food are happier, more productive and more inspiring to those around them.

Well done to all of you for taking the first step and researching the subject of healthy snacks. I want to express a THANK YOU for reaching for my book and giving it a chance. I hope you will enjoy the journey of dehydrating and creating in the kitchen. Allow nature and your own taste buds to inspire you… I promise it will be worth it.

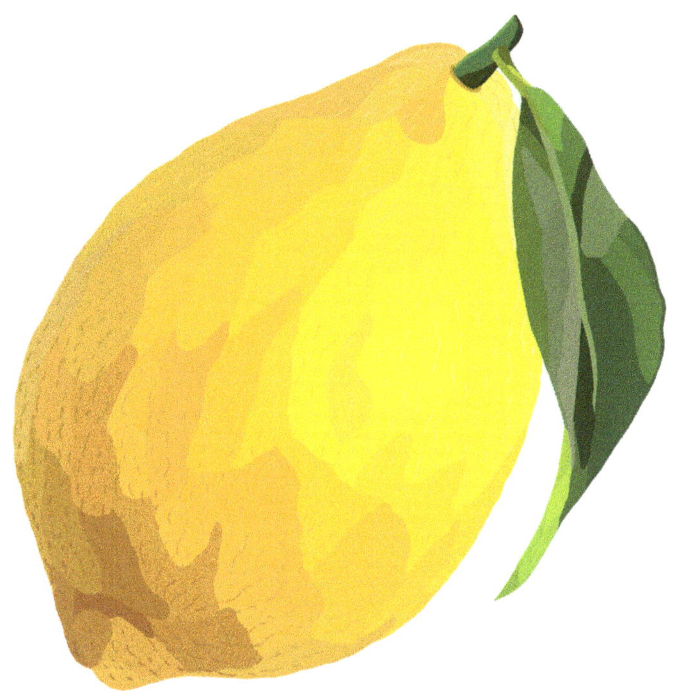

Freezing and Dehydrating to Preserve Food

The original inspiration to start dehydrating fruits and veg came from the surplus of harvesting that I had on my hands each season from my garden. Later on, when I started my 'juicing journey', pulp from juicing vegetables and fruits seemed like great material to use and create something yummy, crunchy, and desirable.

I have to say it: wasting food is UNKIND.

There are too many hungry mouths in this world for any of us to dare to waste food.

Spending more time living in places with people who hardly have enough food on their plates is a lesson I think every human should experience.

Gratitude is always on my mind… Nature is my biggest teacher. In one way or another, one person's surplus is another person's treasure.

If you cannot use all the veg and fruit you have and really cannot share it/freeze it/eat it/compost it, I beg you please do not throw it in the 'regular' bin. Take it to the forest, garden, or any green place and throw it on the soil (without the packaging of course!) Nature will do the rest.

My favorite methods of saving surplus food are freezing and dehydrating.

I… freeze the pulp left over from juicing fruits and veggies we haven't consumed if I'm going to be away from home for a while

… the harvest surplus from my and my neighbor's garden

… buy overripe fruit that's on sale — I can't resist it…

 and I just smile when I find it waiting there in the freezer drawer when I need it the most.

And yes – I freeze some of my crackers if want them to last an extra-long time.

Dehydrating, or drying food is a form of food preservation older than agriculture itself.

Drying made it possible to extend a healthy diet beyond the immediate stages of a fresh kill or a windfall of fresh edible plants. When food is purged of most of its moisture, it no longer provides a good habitat for the strains of bacteria, yeast and molds that can ruin it. Dried food is also lighter and so more portable than moist food, helping to ensure nutrition even as people travelled and explored new territories.

Nowadays it's still a major means of preserving food. Look at rice, seafood, pasta, spices, legumes, grains, fruits, vegetables and meats...

Old processes such as heat/sun and air circulation/wind are still used as well. Is it sunny? Is there a breeze? If so, you have what it takes to dry food, because the Earth's atmosphere is the oldest and largest dehydrator there is.

I believe that after you and your kids have tried some of my recipes you'll want at some point to invest in a reliable dehydrator – it will seem like a natural step.

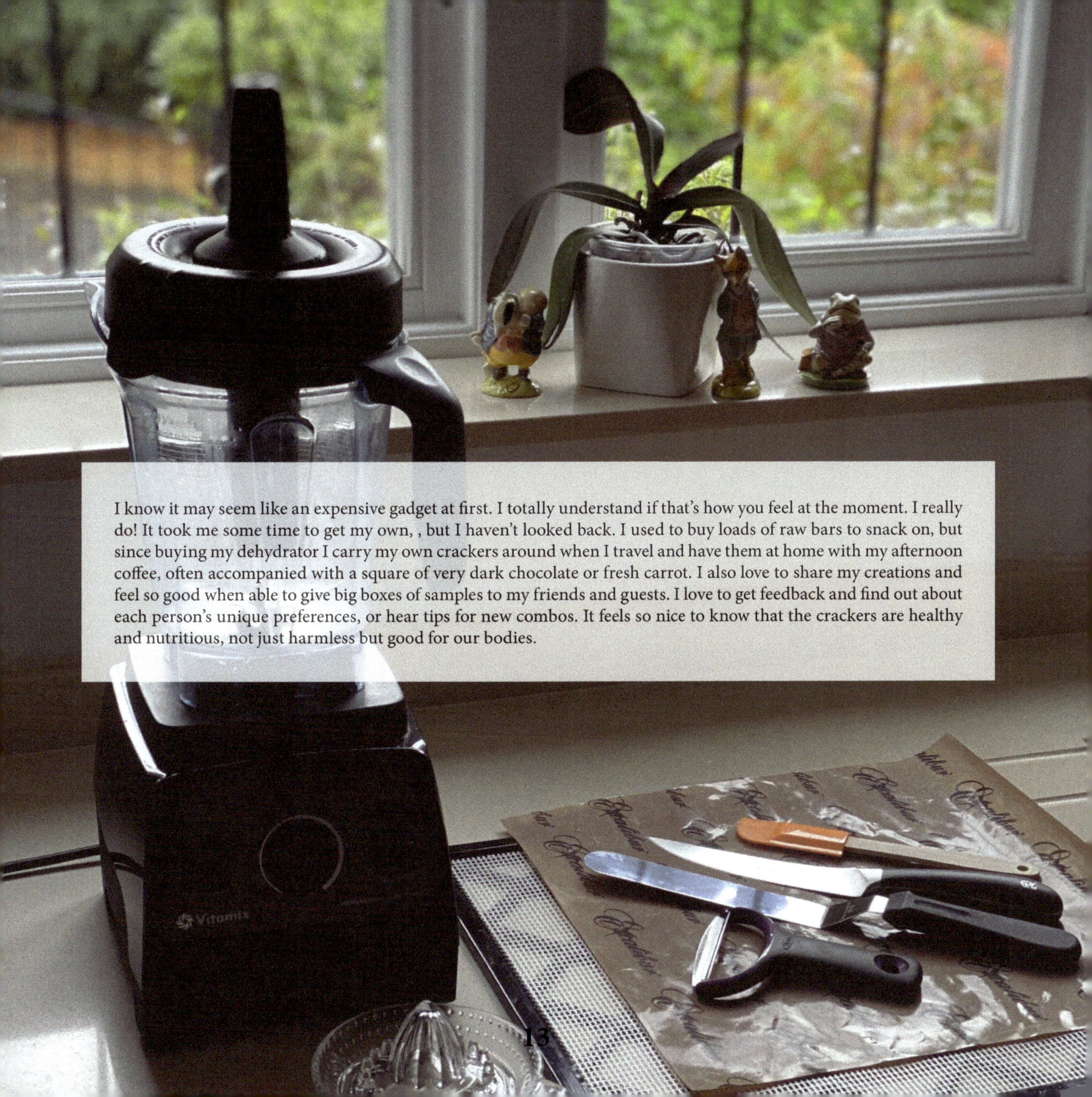

I know it may seem like an expensive gadget at first. I totally understand if that's how you feel at the moment. I really do! It took me some time to get my own, , but I haven't looked back. I used to buy loads of raw bars to snack on, but since buying my dehydrator I carry my own crackers around when I travel and have them at home with my afternoon coffee, often accompanied with a square of very dark chocolate or fresh carrot. I also love to share my creations and feel so good when able to give big boxes of samples to my friends and guests. I love to get feedback and find out about each person's unique preferences, or hear tips for new combos. It feels so nice to know that the crackers are healthy and nutritious, not just harmless but good for our bodies.

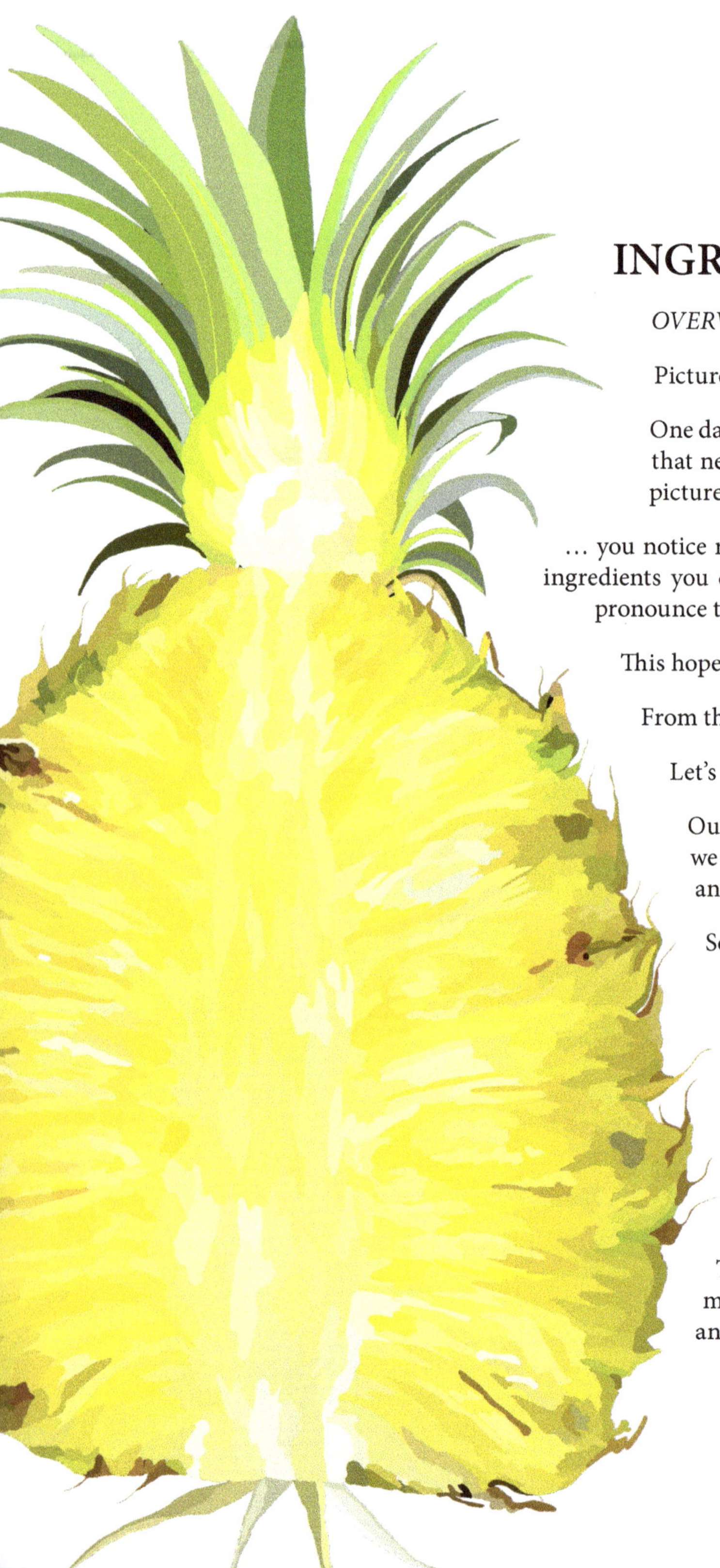

INGREDIENTS

OVERVIEW

Picture this…

One day you feel like trying a new recipe, making some nice new meal, using that new cookbook you've wanted to test for a while. You locate the page/picture in the book which seems like the ONE and…

… you notice recipe after recipe that the ingredients lists are long. Also, there are ingredients you do not have at home, don't even know what they mean or how to pronounce them. Yes, very frustrating…

This hopefully will not happen with my MAD (about crackers) book.

From the very start, I want to assure you that all these recipes are flexible.

Let's build on the ingredients you have in your reach.

Our target is to make something yummy and healthy, and that's what we will get if we use clean, raw, chemically untreated fruits, vegetables, and seeds. And maybe some nuts, spices, and herbs if you wish.

So, what ingredients do I use to make crackers in this book?

Very simply put:

FRUIT

FRESH VEGETABLES

RAW SEEDS, nuts, coconut oil

FLOWERS

The whole point of this book is to make your kids (and yourself) eat more uncooked veggies and fruits in absolutely the most enjoyable and desirable form, possibly on a daily basis.

14

FRUITS AND VEGETABLES

In recipes across this book I use fresh:

Apples, Pears, Bananas, Plums/Prunes, Peaches, Apricots, Pineapples, Oranges, Tangerines, Cherries, Mangos, Lemons, Raspberries, Strawberries, Kiwis, Figs, Papaya, Rhubarb, Yellow Melons, Cranberries.

Carrots, Parsnips, Beetroot, Cauliflowers, Tomatoes, Pumpkins, Butternut Squashes, Broccoli, Bell Peppers, Green Peas, Kale, Spinach, Sprouted Lentils, Sprouted Mung Beans, Garlic, Chives, Spring Onions, Red Onions, Leeks, Celery, Olives, Sprouted Buckwheat (technically a grain).

Some dried fruits: Golden and Brown Raisins, Cranberries, Papaya, Prunes, Figs.

Other goodies (spices, condiments and herbs)- I use in my crackers and couple of them in recipes in this book:

Ginger, Vanilla, Cinnamon, Cocoa powder, Cocoa nibs, Maca powder, Cumin Seeds, Chili, Himalayan Salt, Yeast flakes, Honey, Tahina, Tomato paste, Oregano, Rosemary, Thyme, Turmeric, Mustard seeds, Curry powder, Nutmeg, Garam Masala, Black Pepper, Cardamon, Carob, Dried Baobab Fruit powder, Psyllium husk, sea vegetables (such as Dulse, Nori, Kelp, Kombu etc).

Sourcing:

If you can, try to find clean, organic ingredients so that the end product of our endeavor – the cracker – is actually healthy.

Go preferably for Mother Nature's gifts which are in season and locally grown.

As I have mentioned, the initial spark of my own dream and passion for dehydrating came during those times when I had a surplus of fruit and vegetables in my own and my neighbor's gardens.

I want to encourage you all to start growing your own food. It can become a very rewarding way to teach your kids where the carrot and apple actually come from. Imagine the day when their small hands harvest the strawberries, juicy tomatoes, or cucumbers you planted together.

PARSNIPS

There is something about parsnips...

As you may have noticed (or are soon about to) I use parsnips in crackers quite often.

It is a widely accessible and very affordable vegetable, even in its organic state. It's very easy to grow. It lasts a long time (even months) if stored properly (preferably paper-wrapped and in the fridge.)

It has been cultivated for its sweet roots since ancient times.

It has been even used as a sweetener, before the arrival of cane and beet sugar to Europe.

This humble looking vegetable (which I feel is often overlooked) is incredibly versatile to use in any kitchen: either traditionally or in a 'raw foodie' recipe, like mine.

This edible taproot, which contains only 75 kcal in 100 g can be:

Steamed

Roasted

Boiled

Baked

Puréed

Fried

Even made into wine...

Parsnip makes great baby food, steamed or roasted, and then puréed or cut into soft safe early finger food. I like raw parsnip blended smoothly with a slice of avocado- this delicious combo may be loved by your baby too if you give it a chance.

I find that for me, the best use of all is to turn raw parsnips into varieties of appealing crackers for the whole family.

Parsnips contain a plethora of vitamins (vitamin C, K, A, folate), minerals (such as manganese, phosphorus, potassium, copper...), antioxidants, soluble and insoluble fiber. Try to preserve the skin of this cream-colored root, only peel it finely, or carefully scrub to remove the soil. As we all know the goodies are in the skin.

Possible benefits to the human body include its antioxidant, anti-inflammatory and anti-fungal properties...

Parsnips are: *80% WATER, 18% CARBOHYDRATES - 5% sugars, 5% fiber, 1.2% PROTEIN, 0.3% FAT*

Parsnips are great!

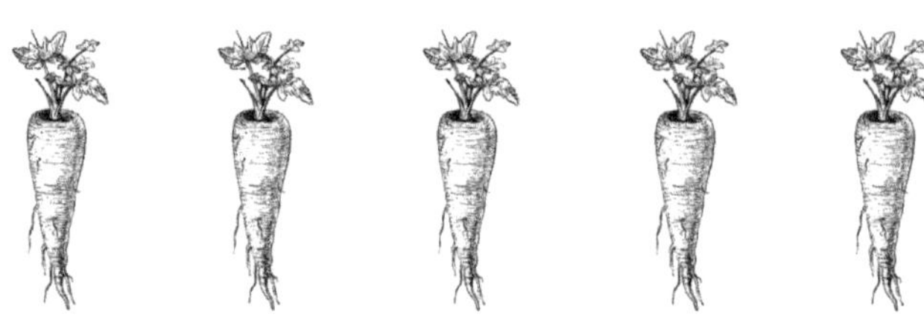

SEEDS AND NUTS

Used in my recipes are raw:

Flax seeds (brown and yellow)	Coconut (mature and whole, if you can't find it, then desiccated shredded coconut is a fine alternative)
Sunflower seeds	Walnuts
Hemp seeds	Keshu
Pumpkin seeds	Almonds
Sesame seeds	Hazel nuts
Chia seeds	
Poppy seeds	

Whenever using nuts in the recipe, you can replace them with seeds of your choice if you have any worries about nut allergies. Feel free to experiment with different seeds and nuts in a specific recipe. Swap and compare different variations.

It is always a good idea to soak seeds and nuts before eating or using in crackers. This may seem like extra work at first, but it is good for you and makes the nuts easier to digest. When soaked, they start to awaken, to live; and this life force will energize your body.

To soak the nuts and seeds, place them into a glass jar or a bowl and cover it with at least double the amount of filtered water. Leave for approx. 6 hours, or overnight.

After soaking, rinse them really well before placing them in a blender. Never use the soaking-water. You can keep them in the fridge until ready to use. (You can also freeze pre-soaked and pre-rinsed nuts to have them ready for use in the future, or if you have a sudden 'urge' to make crackers.)

You can sprout nuts/seeds before using them in the recipe... that's 'upping the game' of a raw and healing way to prepare foods. For the sake of keeping this book simple and the recipes easy to follow and fast to make, check page 20 in this book for "how to" sprout seeds and pulses. For more detailed information about sprouting nuts and grains that is beyond the scope of this book (there are nuances in these processes, hence a little more care is needed) visit www.23blossom.com.

Personally, I prefer to use seeds in my crackers. I consume nuts sparingly.

The analysis of the content and ratio of omega-3 and omega-6 fatty acids in specific seeds and nuts is out of the scope of this recipe book. I think it is quite an important detail to pay attention to, especially if you're vegetarian/vegan and rely on nuts/seeds as a source of fats in your diet, as well as for all of you who enjoy eating nuts more often and in larger amounts. For those who are interested I promise to go into more detail in some of my future blog posts. For now I can't resist but share the little known fact that omega-3 fatty acids can be found in greens (arugula, spinach, brussel sprouts, kale, romain) among which PURSLANE (one of the 'wild edibles') has the highest content.

COCONUT OIL

In all my recipes I do use a spoonful of raw virgin coconut oil. It is kind of a healthy habit at this point. The idea behind this is to add a bit of healthy fat to crackers to enable the body to absorb and use the fat-soluble vitamins from the veggies and fruits. Of course, it is not totally necessary. Feel free to make these recipes your own – if you do not like coconut oil, or really want to prepare very low-fat crackers, skip the coconut oil. Adding raw seeds/nuts to crackers already means having some fats there anyway.

I believe healthy fats in a daily diet are necessary for our wellbeing. I personally eat between half to a whole avocado a day and add freshly grounded flax seeds to my salad. A variety of raw seeds added to crackers will provide an array of healthy fats, minerals, and vitamins necessary for your kids' healthy growth, development, and overall energy. They need this to run around and play!

One more reason for adding the coconut oil: it is a secret trick to make your crackers or dried fruit slices even more crunchy. You can try and test it yourself! If we store crackers in the fridge, the temperature makes the coconut oil become solid, and that hardens the cracker even more which adds up to the overall sensation and experience of lovely CRISPY-CRUNCHINESS.

Raw nuts and seeds are protein and healthy fat staples in my kitchen. Some are higher in oils than others and go rancid faster. If you're like me and shop for them in bulk, store them in glass jars in the fridge or freezer.

In raw food stores, one can find crackers based on raw seeds and maybe with salt/some spices. If you like seeded crackers like those, try to recreate the same at home. Maybe adding little extras such as sun-dried tomatoes or pitted chopped olives is worth trying. Or a piece of fresh veg for that matter such as bell peppers, beetroot, onion etc.

When wet, flaxseeds or chia seeds become gelatinous in consistency and bind together, which makes a mix that can be spread across your dehydrator tray. In all our crackers they serve as a binding agent along with sticky fruit (such as ripe bananas, ripe mangos, ripe apricots, ripe figs, etc). In this book I am focusig on recipes that contain whole fruits/vegetables along with seeds. Margo's crackers are lighter in texture, have natural flavor, color and better overall balanced fat/carb/fiber content ratio than if they were only made of seeds.

SWEETENERS

If any at all I prefer to use:

DATES

They are rich in fiber, potassium, thiamin, riboflavin, niacin, vitamin B6, iron, magnesium, pantothenic acid.

OTHER DRIED FRUITS such as apricots, figs, raisins, mangos, prunes... I soak them for at least a couple of hours before making crackers, as they may contain sulfur and possibly dust and dirt etc. (some dry fruit sold in stores is dried outdoors in the sun when mass-produced) ...

HONEY

If possible, aim to buy and use raw (non-pasteurized) local organic honey. Bees make honey from the nectar of flowering plants. It is a gift from nature, quite a miraculous substance overall. Raw honey has medicinal benefits, contains minerals, enzymes, B-complex vitamins, etc. To be considered raw, the honey must not have been heated during the extraction process. Note! It is unsafe for babies younger than 12-18 months to eat honey as it can contain spores that cause botulism. Honey also adds a wonderful, sweet aroma to the crackers: I like it especially in my 'floral' recipes.

STEVIA

Maybe grow your own Stevia plants on your windowsill and use its leaves.

AGAVE syrup, raw and organic.

Sprouts and SPROUTING

In some of the recipes I use sprouts, so I want to take time and explain why I think it's worth spending a couple of minutes for a few days to get your sprouts growing and ready for cracker preparation. It is quite simple, and I promise after a couple of attempts the process of sprouting will become second nature to you. To me it is a daily habit now – to rinse and take care of my sprouts every day. It literally does take a couple of minutes. The health benefits of incorporating sprouts into crackers or, in fact, in many other different ways into your family meals are huge…

Seeds are the very essence of life

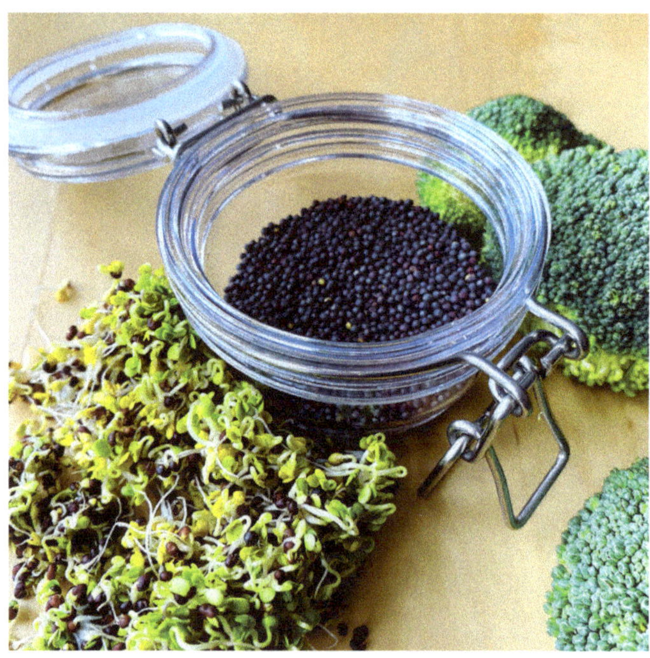

All the energy and life of plants goes towards making seeds.

Each seed holds vitamins, protein, fats, minerals, and carbohydrates (starches) in reserve, waiting for a suitable environment to begin growing.

During the process of sprouting – starches (complex carbohydrates) are transformed by the action of enzymes into simple sugars.

Complex proteins are converted into simple amino acids.

Fats are changed into fatty acids.

All these are substances our bodies easily digest.

Vitamin C is produced in larger amounts during sprouting. As well as vitamin A, B complex, E, U…

Seeds contain some minerals, and while 'waking up' and growing they absorb minerals from the water they've soaked in. An example of sprouts containing extra high levels of calcium is SESAME. There is loads of potassium in sunflower/sesame/mung/almond sprouts, iron in alfalfa/fenugreek/lentils/adzuki/mung bean sprouts…

Only uncooked germinated seeds/grains/nuts can give us **'living energy'**. (Try to plant cooked beans… will they grow?)

Please do not cook your sprouts if you want the healing benefits! The life energy in fresh sprouts stimulates the body's inherent self-cleansing and self-healing abilities.

HOW:

Choose the seeds you want to sprout. Maybe start with easy ones (lentils, mungo…) A variety of seeds can be easily grown to eat as sprouts, for example: RADISH, BROCOLLI, ALFALFA, LENTILS, MUNGO, ADZUKI, PEA, CHICKPEA, FENUGREEK, SUNFLOWER, SESAME, or even grains (BUCKWHEAT, RYE, WILD RICE, QUINOA, KAMUT) and some nuts for those with a little more experience.

Place the seeds in a glass jar (approx. 1/5 of the jar volume) or, as we like to measure, 2 handfuls. Then fill the jar with filtered water to SOAK at room temperature. Secure the sprouting mesh over the jar. (Have a look at my blog to see what I mean by 'sprouting mesh' or simply use a strainer to stop the seeds from running away from you while you rinse them.)

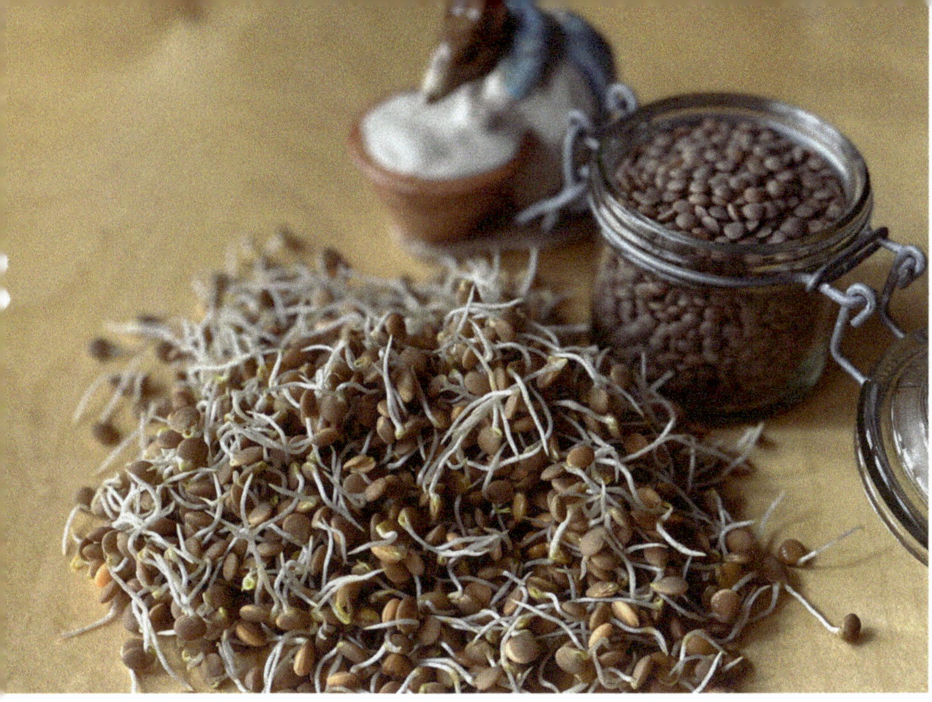

After soaking the seeds for approx. 10-12 hours rinse them very well and drain all the water from the jar. The seeds should remain damp, but with no water left. Shake if you need to. (This is where your sprouting mesh comes in handy - I made my own, it is not difficult- you can create one too). Repeat the rinsing at least every 12 hours, (drain very well each time) until the sprouts are ready, usually about 2-4 days.

In warmer climates, bacteria grow faster, so please rinse more often. It is important to rinse!

Bacteria growth could ruin your sprouts and make you unwell! Feel free to turn the jars upside down between the rinses, sideways, or at a slight angle while stored up-side-down on the side of an empty bowl... Eat the sprouts straight away or keep in the fridge for several days (up to 1 week) and of course use them in different cracker recipes.

Once the sprouts are stored in the fridge, no rinsing is required. Just rinse before you eat them or before starting to prepare crackers. I think they are great to use in SALADS, VEGGIE BURGERS, WRAPS and ROLLS, SANDWICHES, SMOOTHIES, DIPS, and SPREADS, STIRFRIES, HEALTHY BAKING, SOUPS, and raw DEHYDRATED CRACKERS (my favorites!)

If the sprouts grow too fast, and you can't use them all, you can freeze them for future yummy crackers.

Warning Kidney beans are dangerous to eat raw and undercooked, so should never be eaten sprouted ****

SPROUTING is an amazingly easy way to grow fresh healthy vitamins, minerals, and enzyme-rich greens anywhere, anytime, all year round. I am passionate about living a healthy and happy life and making sprouting happen in more and more joyful homes. Some facts about the great benefits: they are a superhealthy addition to your plate, high in fiber, vitamins, proteins, essential fatty acids, minerals, they help digestion, weight loss, pH balance in the human body... Low in calories and glycaemic index (compared to unsprouted seeds and pulses) and much easier to digest. Fresh, crunchy, even spicy... And they all have unique tastes.

I utilize sprouts only in a couple of my chosen-for-the-book recipes. For you the sky is the limit here! Use your inner cracker wizard and create your own cracker combos which include all sorts of sprouted seeds/pulses/nuts.

Nutritional value, raw food, fiber, CALORIES

Did you see the list of ingredients? All are natural, clean and pure foods.

FRUITS AND VEGETABLES ARE GOOD FOR US, as they have lots of vitamins, minerals, and micronutrients.

I think in general, with all the information easily accessible in recent years, the public has become wiser. Consumers are learning to avoid products that contain artificial flavors, artificial colors, and shelf-life extending chemical substances.

Why try to source organic products?

The simplified definition of ORGANIC FOOD – as food grown/produced without conventional pesticides, fertilizers made with synthetic ingredients or sewage sludge, and processed without bioengineering and ionizing radiation- answers the question...

"Scary things" such as pesticides, synthetics, sewage sludge, bioengineering, radiation are not what I want near my body or plate...

Why and how "RAW"?

By raw food, we generally mean food which has not been heated above 104-118°Fahrenheit (40-48°C). This limit on heating is set because higher temperatures start to bring about undesirable changes in the composition of food. Dehydrating of plant-based food by low temperatures warms up and dries the food without destroying most of the natural enzymes (although some are still destroyed). As with everything in the field of nutrition, there continues to be a debate about nitty-gritty details such as the exact temperatures which are safe for preserving enzymes and vitamins in fruits, vegetables, and herbs.

I would suggest that we make it simple.

I decided myself the temperature I am happy to settle with and feel good about. I usually set my dehydrator to 113°Fahrenheit (45°C) to preserve as much natural healing energy in crackers as possible.

If you are in a hurry to finish drying your crackers and, once in a while, pander to that by setting the temperature a little higher, it's not the end of the world.

See this little chart for easy temperature conversion:

Process	Fahrenheit	Celsius
Freeze Water	32	0
Room Temperarture	68	20
Boil Water	212	100

Celsius	Fahrenheit
40.00	104
40.55	105
41.11	106
41.66	107
42.22	108
42.77	109
43.33	110
43.89	111
44.44	112
45.00	113
45.56	114
46.11	115
46.68	116
47.22	117
47.78	118

Energy Content and Calorie Counting

I personally do not count calories. I am aware of the calorie value of foods I am eating now as well as those I have not touched in the last two decades. Over time I learned to listen to and trust my body, observe how my body felt after certain foods, what amounts of food were ticking all the boxes, how often I eat, timing around the clock relative to circadian rhythms, etc. This is also dependent on the season of the year, the place I found myself on the globe with its climate and local produce, the intensity of my work and workouts. Are things I am focused on at that moment more creative, involving the mind such as writing, reading, studying, or more physical, such as gardening, DIY, house redecorating? I want to eat to feel satisfied but not too full. Learn to be a little more conscious and acknowledge the feeling of hunger when it comes. I'm grateful for that self-awareness and recognition of the contrast between feeling hungry and almost full, as well as for the hunger itself. It's good to know that when I finally eat some food, it is because I get a signal from my body that it is actually hungry, not just thirsty, or wants to eat because of habit or social situations.

It will be different for everyone, and I kind of got carried away in the above lines. What I want to say is this: I realize there are people who like to keep count of calories and wish to know the exact numbers.

For those people, I decided to include this very simple calorie chart.

As the recipes are very flexible, and the size of fruits and veggies can differ a lot, knowing the exact calorie content of a specific cracker based on recipes in this book is totally possible but it will take a little mathematical homework!

Here is a tip for how one can go about it:

Weigh the exact amount of individual fruits, vegetables, seeds and nut ingredients you want to use, then multiply each individually by calorie/kJ content per 100g/1oz. Count the total sum of calories/kJ of all ingredients used. (I include both metrics in the chart.)

If you try to make your crackers even in size and divide the total calorie content of ingredients used for a batch by the number of crackers made… there you have it! Calories (or kJ) per cracker.

Another more exact way to get the calorie/kJ content count: once the crackers are dried to your liking, get the total weight of the dry crackers and then you can divide the total calories by the weight. You will get the number of calories per 100g/1oz.

*Do you want to give it a try? Continue to page 29...

In general, I would say it would be lazy and hypocritical of me to try to put the calories as well as exact minerals and vitamins content of cracker and adhere to it, because:

1. I want to keep recipes simple, and would rather say 2-3 apples, 1-2 bananas instead of an exact weight… I would have to be too exact to feel good about my cracker calorie charts. Would I say 100 g of peeled bananas? Or unpeeled? Which exact variety of pears, tomatoes, mangos did I use? That may make crackering not fun at all.

2. Fruits and vegetables differ in size, but not only that – they are all available in different varieties, which can themselves differ in sweetness, water content, color (that means pigments and that translates into micronutrients and antioxidants etc.) … where the tree grew really affects what the fruit contains. Was it a hot summer this year in this place, or just so-so? Is the garden on the hill or in the valley? What is the soil like in the region? Did the fruit ripen naturally? Or did it ripen on the airplane while being imported from other continents? Was the vegetable growing in rested soil, where the crops were rotated? Or in depleted soil somewhere in a big greenhouse? Maybe they were hydroponically grown? Or under clear skies and in a beautiful natural garden with weeds living in harmony with crops we try to grow. Was the crop harvested just this morning or days/weeks ago and stored (how and where). All this and so much more contributes significantly to the content of vitamins, minerals, enzymes, and believe it or not, to the polysaccharides/calories in the fruits and vegetables we eat. So, when I was asked by my friends to estimate the calorie content in cracker recipes I immediately knew that I may not really satisfy some of them. Better to turn this matter into a little scientific project or quest for the reader, instead of giving straight answers – and make you think about all these aspects of the life of plants and the story behind each beautiful piece of fruit and majestic vegetable which ends up on your plate and in your crackers.

In general, what really does make the crackers more calorific is the amount of nuts and seeds used, and its ratio to the fruits and vegetables you decide to use.

... oh, and, of course, the FIBER...

An invaluable bit of info I want to bring up is that FIBER content in all these cracker recipes is very high. Fiber helps slow down the release of sugar into the blood and helps clean our bodies.

Eating foods that contain a substantial amount of fiber helps us eliminate wastes quickly. Wastes allowed to remain too long in the digestive system feed harmful bacteria. Fiber acts like a broom, sweeping the whole digestive system free of circulatory waste and dead cells.

1 pound = 453.6 grams

1 ounce = 28.35 grams

16 ounces = 1 pound

Food stuff	Kilojoules per 100g	Kilojoules per 1g	Calories per 100g	Calories per 1g	Kilojoules per 1oz	Calories per 1oz
1. Vegetables						
Beetroot	184	1.84	44	0.44	52	12
Bellpepper green	117	1.17	28	0.28	33	8
Buckwheat dried	1,440	14.00	343	3.43	397	97
Buckwheat sprouted	716	7.16	179	1.79	204	51
Butternut Squash	167	1.67	40	0.4	47	11
Carrots	146	1.46	35	0.35	41	10
Cauliflower	96	0.96	23	0.23	27	7
Celery	67	0.67	16	0.16	19	5
Chives	126	1.26	30	0.3	36	9
Garlic	623	6.23	149	1.49	177	42
Kale	145	1.45	35	0.35	41	10
Leek	255	2.55	61	0.61	72	17
Lentils dried	1,470	14.70	352	3.52	418	100
Lentils sprouted	444	4.44	106	1.06	125	30
Mung Beans dried	1,450	1.45	347	3.47	411	98
Mung Beans (fully) Sprouted	126	1.26	30	0.3	36	8.5
Olives	339 - 609	3.39 - 6.09	81 - 145	.81 - 1.45	96 - 172	23 - 41
Parsnips	297	2.97	71	0.71	84	20
Pumpkin	84	0.84	20	0.2	24	6
Red Onion	184	1.84	44	0.44	52	12
Spinach	96	0.96	23	0.23	27	7
Spring Onion	133	1.33	32	0.32	38	9
Tomatoes	75	0.75	18	0.18	21	5

Food stuff	Kilojoules per 100g	Kilojoules per 1g	Calories per 100g	Calories per 1g	Kilojoules per 1oz	Calories per 1oz
2. Fruits						
Apples (dep. on the variety)	105 - 217	1.05 - 2.17	25 - 52	.25 - .52	30 - 62	7.1 - 15
Apricots	201	2.01	48	0.48	57	14
Bananas	372	3.72	89	0.89	105	25
Cherries	264	2.64	63	0.63	75	18
Cranberries	192	1.92	46	0.46	54	13
Figs	310	3.10	74	0.74	88	21
Kiwis	255	2.55	61	0.61	72	17
Lemons	121	1.21	29	0.29	34	8
Mangos	251	2.51	60	0.6	71	17
Oranges	205	2.05	49	0.49	58	14
Papayas	180	1.80	43	0.43	51	12
Peaches	163	1.63	39	0.39	46	11
Pears	238	2.38	57	0.57	67	16
Pineapple	209	2.09	50	0.5	59	14
Plums	192	1.92	46	0.46	54	13
Raspberries	218	2.18	52	0.52	62	15
Rhubarb	88	0.88	21	0.21	25	6
Strawberries	134	1.34	32	0.32	38	9
Tangerines	222	2.22	53	0.53	63	15
Yellow Melon	142	1.42	34	0.34	40	10
3. Raw Seeds						
Chia seeds	2,033	20.33	486	4.86	576	138
Flax seeds	2,234	22.34	534	5.34	633	151
Hemp seeds	2,313	23.13	553	5.53	655	157
Poppy seeds	2,197	21.97	525	5.25	622	149
Pumpkin seeds	2,340	23.40	559	5.59	652	158
Sesame seeds	2,363	23.63	565	5.65	669	160
Sunflower seeds	2,440	24.40	504	5.04	692	166

Food stuff	Kilojoules per 100g	Kilojoules per 1g	Calories per 100g	Calories per 1g	Kilojoules per 1oz	Calories per 1oz
4. Raw Nuts						
Almonds	2,502	25.02	598	5.98	709	170
Cashew	2,402	24.02	574	5.74	681	163
Coconut (raw oil)	3,732	37.32	892	8.92	1058	253
Coconut (meat raw mature)	1,481	14.81	354	3.54	419	100
Hazelnut	2,702	27.02	646	6.46	766	183
Macadamias	3,004	30.04	718	7.18	851	204
Peanuts	2,372	23.72	567	5.67	927	161
Pecans	2,891	28.91	691	6.91	819	196
Pine nuts	2,815	28.15	673	6.73	798	191
Pistachio	2,380	23.80	569	5.69	674	161
Walnut	2,736	27.36	654	6.54	775	184
5. Dried Fruit						
Apricots	1,008	10.08	241	2.41	285	68
Cranberries	1,288	12.88	308	3.08	365	87
Dates	1,160	11.60	277	2.77	329	79
Dessicated Coconut (meat)	2,760	27.60	660	6.6	782	187
Figs	1,041	10.41	249	2.49	295	71
Golden Sultanas	1,263	12.63	302	3.02	358	86
Mangos	1,334	13.34	319	3.19	378	90
Papayas	1,079	10.79	258	2.58	306	73
Plums dried (prunes)	1,004	10.04	240	2.4	285	68
Raisins	1,251	12.51	299	2.99	355	85

		A	B	C
	Food Item	**Weight of food item (grams or ounces)**	**Calories/kJ of this ingredient per g/oz**	**Multiply column A x B = C**
1				
2				
3				
4				
5				
6				
7				
8				
9				
10				
Value E = the total calories/kJ of all ingredients in your blender added together:				

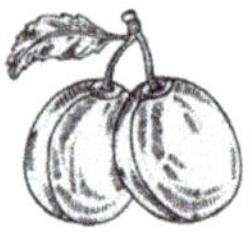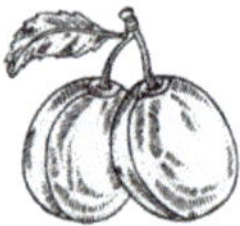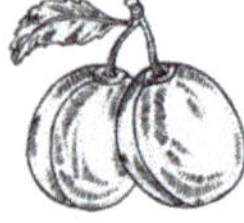

- **value A** = real weight of the individual food item used
- **value B** = cal/kJ per weight unit (g/oz) in the individual food item- find it in the charts on pages 25,26,27

  *I sourced these values from a couple of official sources & I tried my best to average them (for my use and yours)
- **value C** = cal/kJ per singular ingredient (real amount) used
- **value E** = cal/kJ per all ingredients (real amount) used

Calories Counting FUN Mathematical EXERCISE :

- Prior to placing all ingredients into the blender, weigh each ingredient and note it as value 'A' in this simple chart. (column A)

- Look up calories/kJ of each ingredient used (pages 25,26,27) -and note down the value as number '**B**' in this same chart. (column B)

- Multiply the values in columns A and B to get value '**C**' (column C)- which represents the amount of calories/kJ contained in each singular ingredient used to make this unique batch of crackers.

- Now add up all the **C**'s to get the value '**E**' (value $E = C1+C2+C3+C4$.....etc). Value '**E**' represents the real calories/kJ contained in the blender once all the ingredients are placed in it. (i.e. the total energy content in all the ingredients used for this batch of crackers)

- Once your crackers are fully and properly dehydrated -> WEIGH the whole BATCH -> this is value '**D**'.

- The final step is to divide: $E \div D = T$ ->   to understand how many cal/kJ are contained in 100g/1oz of crackers you just made. (the number you get is actually the real calorie content in the crackers in this particular batch). I named it value 'T'.

Enough? Or shall we take this fun maths exercise one step further:

In order to estimate cal/kJ content in 1 singular cracker:

- Count how many crackers are in the batch: '**N**' is number of all crackers in this batch. Divide $E \div N = S$

- '**S**' is the calorie/kJ content in one singular cracker in this specific batch.

***This is far from a precise way of getting the exact one-cracker-calories-content unless you manage to make your crackers EQUAL in weight. (Could say 'size' too if you were precise enough about thickness when spreading your blended cracker mix before scoring it and as well very precise scoring it into equally sized shaped crackers).**

As I recommend in the chapter 'The perfect cracker' on page 42 - the same applies here- make written notes when crackering, creating, weighing and measuring. Possibly start your own 'CRACKER JOURNAL' to gather and note down your favourite recipes, ratios, all important observations, etc

Hope I made you smile! ☺

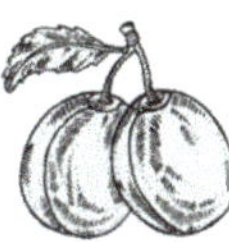

- value D = real weight of the whole batch of fully dried crackers
- value T = cal/kJ per weight unit (g/oz) of final product (crackers)
- value N = number (how many) of crackers you made in this whole batch
- value S = cal/kJ in 1 cracker

Utensils and Equipment

Sharp knife

Fruit peeler

Chopping board

Big bowl

Spatula

Blender

Dehydrator

Dehydrator sheets

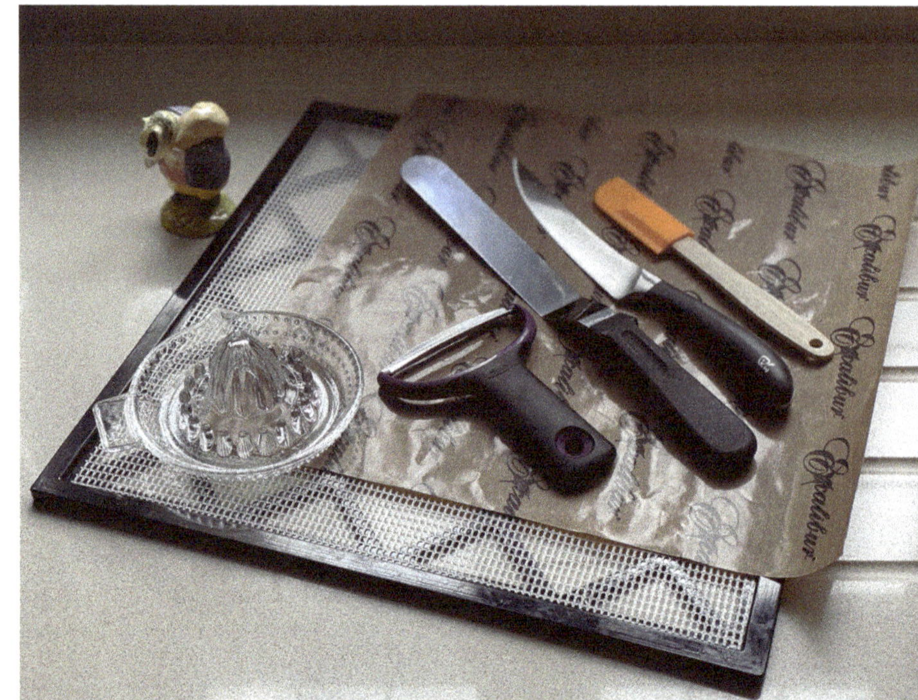

BLENDER

I personally think a good blender is a must in a kitchen where healthy nutrition is a priority. I use mine every day. For inspiration I will mention examples of what my blender does for me:

Green juices

Smoothies

Frozen desserts (instant ice-creams & sorbets)

Soups (cold and warm as well as hot)

Dips, sauces, dressings

Nut/seed milk

Nuts/seeds/sprouted grains flours

Nut/seed butters

Pulverizing dried herbs (eg. making green protein powders or spice blends)

Crushing ice

Chopping veggies (for salads etc.)

… and, of course, CRACKER PREPARATION

As you can see, I want to spend as little time preparing my food as necessary, so I let my blender do all the work.

Which BLENDER to Choose?

Hmmm…

I want to be as honest as I can here.

I lived and worked in quite a number of households and kitchens with their varying appliances. As you can imagine I came across and used different types/brands of blenders. Saying that I fully realize I am no expert on reviewing blenders nor dehydrators. I'm equally sure there are many more I haven't come across yet.

So, all I can say is I am more than happy with the blender I own now – which is a *Vitamix*. I love it! (I can imagine my husband's smiles when he reads this...) I also have a *NUTRIBULLET*, which comes in handy when in need of a quick smoothie or iced coffee for one etc.

Vitamix is my 'go-to' when it comes to cracker preparation. For many, many reasons. One of them is the tamper – it really helps to blend solid biomass with not too much water added to a blend. I will review in more detail my experience with a *Vitamix* on my blog for those who are interested. This book wants to be about healthy crackers and the joy which comes from creating them and sharing them, not about the kitchen appliances.

DEHYDRATOR SHEETS

These are dehydrator tray liners that play a vital part in dehydrating crackers and other goodies. They protect the dehydrator trays, mesh, and the dehydrator itself from sticky messes and make the peeling of the final dry product (crackers, fruit leathers, etc) easy, fast and convenient. Unlike dehydrator meshes and trays, the sheets usually DO NOT come with the dehydrator and need to be purchased separately. It is worthwhile investing in good quality, durable, non-stick, reusable silicone sheets, which are safe to use. The original Excalibur dehydrator sheets are made of a material called Paraflexx. You may come across words such as Teflex, Teflon, silicone, or ultra-silicone when doing your shopping research. After purchase, while waiting for them to be delivered, you can improvise and use parchment paper instead. Good quality dehydrator sheets are easy to clean. Simply wipe them clean with warm water. Once in a while, I place mine in the dishwasher. Remember to dry them well before storing them.

DEHYDRATOR

You can try your first dehydrating experiments in your oven, setting it to the lowest possible temperature, preferably with the fan on if your oven has that feature. After gaining some experience you may want to invest in a home dehydrator. What is a DEHYDRATOR? Simply put, it is a kitchen gadget combining a circulating fan with a heating element to heat food from approximately 95 to 165°F (35-74°C). What's inside dehydrators? They have several layered trays made of plastic or metal that allow warm air to circulate around the food, so the food dries evenly.

The main reason to go for one is to have more control over dehydrating (temperature, time) and nice, even predictable, results. Of course, it depends on which one you opt for but I dare to say that with my personal

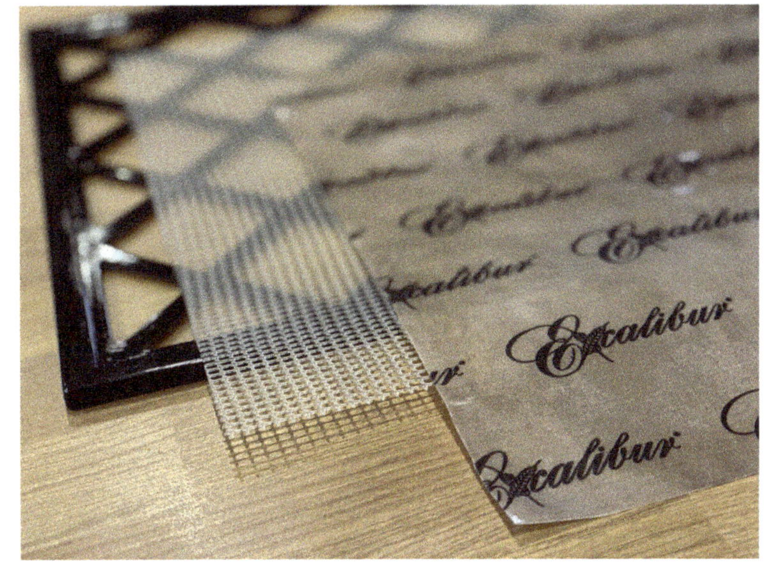

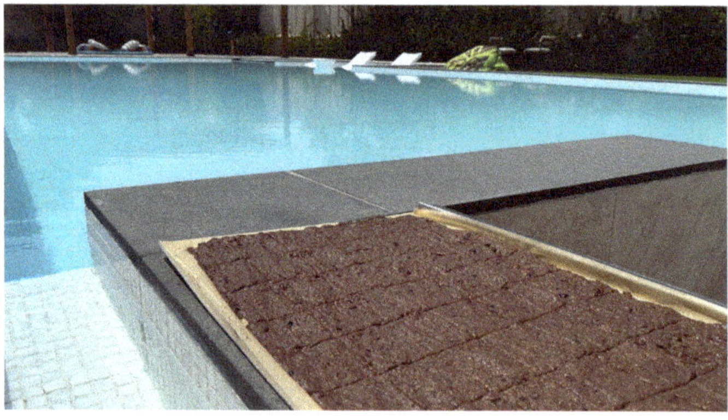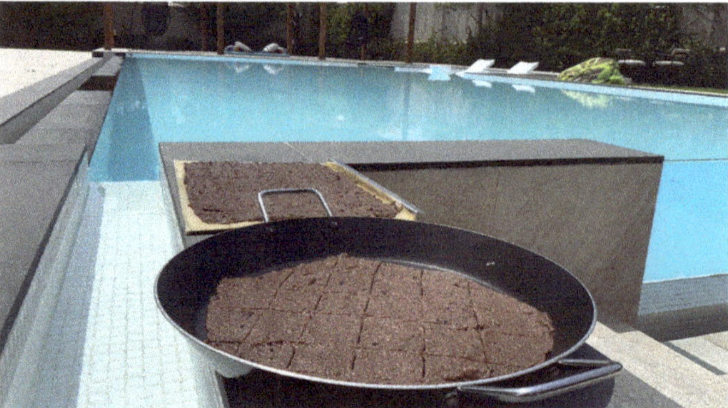

*my attempt to dry crackers in the desert SUN

choice less energy is consumed in drying the crackers or any food really compared to drying in the oven: an extra bonus.

Regarding dehydrators, I will take the liberty to share some tips here.

I took a long time to research my options before I invested in my first and for now only dehydrator. I own an **Excalibur** with nine trays, a timer, and temperature-setting rotating buttons. I'm very happy with the way it functions.

It dries the cracker mix evenly; it is not too noisy...

Other brands (I noticed they exist but so far haven't had a chance to try or use them) are:

Tribest Sedona
Stockli
Brod & Taylor
Cabela's
Weston
Nesco
Lem
Avantco
I'm sure there are many more out there.

Choosing a Dehydrator:

Before jumping in with the first dehydrator that someone recommends, do a little research. You will save yourself some time, frustration and hopefully money!

Here are some simple rules of thumb for purchasing a dehydrator:

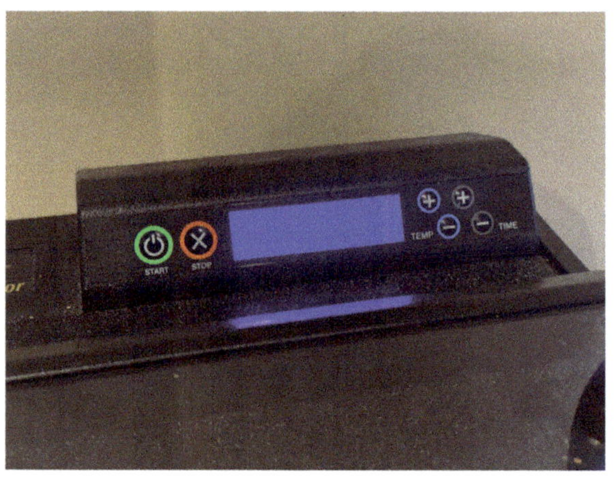

Budget

Your budget is maybe the biggest factor, as the prices vary a lot. Of course, there may be some good machines in the lower price ranges but there are definitely some great ones if you have a few more dollars/pounds/euros to spend. I think the easiest way to get what you want is to ASK SANTA THIS YEAR! Or – if you have time and patience – to scour garage sales, thrift shops, charity shops, online marketplaces on Facebook, Craigslist, Gumtree, eBay, etc. You may find the "one for you" there. Also, check the manufacturers' websites or get their newsletters to be reminded of sales and coupons. Look for lightning deals on Amazon, you may find refurbished or return models which can be certified and hold the same or similar warranty. Check Amazon's warehouse.

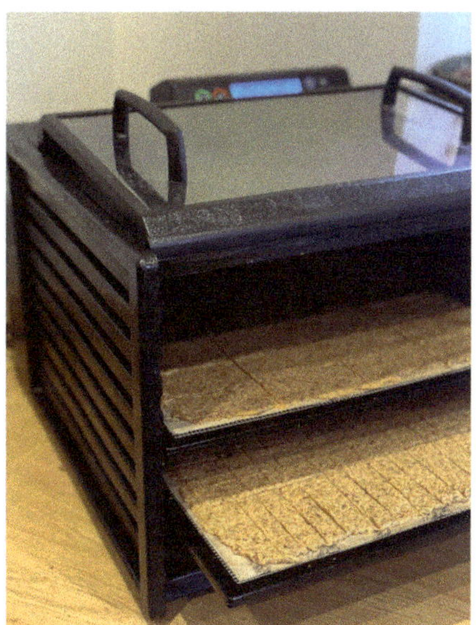

Try to ask friends if they have one they never use and if they would mind you testing your first recipes with it. (Maybe for some free delicious crackers in exchange?)

This may be a great way for you to try making crackers first before spending money on a dehydrator with features you really want!

Remember as well: the worst dehydrator is the one you don't use.

Temperature Adjustment

Temperature adjustment is a vital feature of a dehydrator. It allows you to change the temperature for different types of foods. The sky is the limit, especially if you decide to experiment with other drying culinary endeavors apart from crackers.

Machines that have a simple on/off switch are usually single temperature machines. They are of a fixed temperature that may or may not be safe enough to do raw meat/fish drying, for example.

Timer

A lot of dehydrators come with a simple on/off switch which is fine when you want to keep a close eye on the drying process. I personally want to load the unit up and forget about it. I think a model with a built-in timer is a great choice. It makes it easy to dry foods overnight without over-drying them and wasting energy.

Wattage

Get the most you can afford. A 250-watt machine will take too long to dry those things that need longer drying times. It wastes energy and costs you more in electricity in the long run. Wattage varies per machine, so make sure to compare it as well as price and settle on the amount you can afford. (Of course, more wattage means more initial electricity usage, but you will have to balance that with a lower wattage machine having to run longer for the same results.)

There are basically two types of fans:

Horizontal fans work from front to back across all trays. Think the 'slide-in trays machine' like the Excalibur.

Pros: the airflow affects all trays at the same time across the food, and you can make full use of the tray. This is the most efficient form of dehydrating.

Cons: rotation may still be needed for long drying times with fruits, as airflow still concentrates mostly in the middle trays at the back of the machine. They tend to be more expensive and larger.

Vertical fans have stackable trays with a fan on the top unit or the bottom base unit. There is usually an open channel for upflow created with center holes in each tray.

Pros: many of these can be stacked with additional trays to expand your drying.

Cons: not as efficient as the horizontal trays and need to be rotated during use. Each tray has a hole in the middle to help with airflow, hence a reduction in how much you can get on a tray.

Ultimately, a good machine that has a strong motor will work for you regardless. I personally prefer the horizontal fan as per all the pros mentioned above, as well as the fact that I can remove any tray at any time without the need to move all the trays.

Trays

Skip the 4- or 5-tray machines that you cannot add to. You will lose half of those while doing anything like greens (kale crisps for example) as you have to make extra room. Go for expandable vertical trays or 7+ tray horizontal machines.

Construction

One way that the inexpensive machines keep the cost down is to cut back on the material used. The trays are made from flimsy plastic that can be broken easily when handling. It is usually a clear polycarbonate that will be quite fragile. Another downside to a low-cost machine is that many of them will have a tray that warps from the heat of the fan.

You want a machine with trays that are made from sturdy plastic or stainless steel, that do not feel they will crack at the slightest touch.

Stainless versus Plastic: This is a personal preference. The plastics used in most modern dehydrators are BPA-free, but you will want to do your due diligence – read the manufacturers' specifications on any machine you want to use. Be sure to look at not only the cabinet construction but also at the construction of the trays when making your decision.

Space

Know the space you have to store a dehydrator when in use and out of use. Look not only at where you will use it, but also where you will store it when not in use. Do you have a spot in the garage you can spare? Or a closet where it can stay during those seasons that you are not using it? Consider all of the dimensions of the unit – top to bottom, front to back, and side to side – to make sure it's going to fit in the spot you've chosen.

Noise Levels

The truth is that every dehydrator makes some noise when running.

Unfortunately, there are not many things that you can do to the dehydrator itself to help muffle the noise it creates. You don't want to impede the fan in any fashion, nor make it so that the vents can't completely vent out moisture.

Still, there are a couple of tips that can help to reduce the noise:

Place it in a room that you are not in. Maybe a clean garage, separate room, hallway, etc... We have ours in the front of the house in a utility room.

Place a thin towel or mat underneath a dehydrator to stop vibrations against a hard surface. Don't make it so thick that it impedes performance. Be careful though if the machine has vents on the underside – a piece of cardboard is your best bet if you absolutely need to control it.

Use a barrier. Just like a closed door, placing something between you and the dehydrator to help muffle the sound a little.

MAKING CRACKERS: How It's Done

Place all the ingredients in a food processor and mix well, adding just enough water to create a spreadable consistency. While blending use the tamper; it makes blending easier, especially if you try to make your mixture NOT too runny. Tampers assist blending the mass more evenly and helps to keep your blender engine safe. Recipes based on very soft fruits and vegetables such as berries, peaches, mango, melon, tomatoes etc. may not require adding water to the blend at all, as the water content in these fruits/veg is very high and they are naturally very easy to blend. If you think the recipe still needs some water to enable safe blending, pour some into the blender, but only a small amount, and add more only if necessary. Avoid having your blender totally full. Blending is easier when the blender is just half to 2/3 full. If you find yourself in a situation where your blender jug is too small or the total amount of ingredients you want to use in a specific recipe doesn't fit in the blender, simply divide all the ingredients in their corresponding ratios and blend in two 'half-batches' instead. Another possible way to deal with your blender having a smaller jug is simply proportionally reducing the amount of the ingredients suggested in the recipe (especially if you're only testing the recipes for the first time).

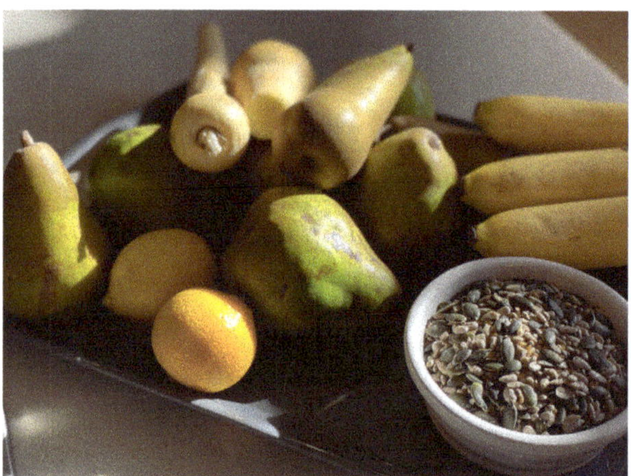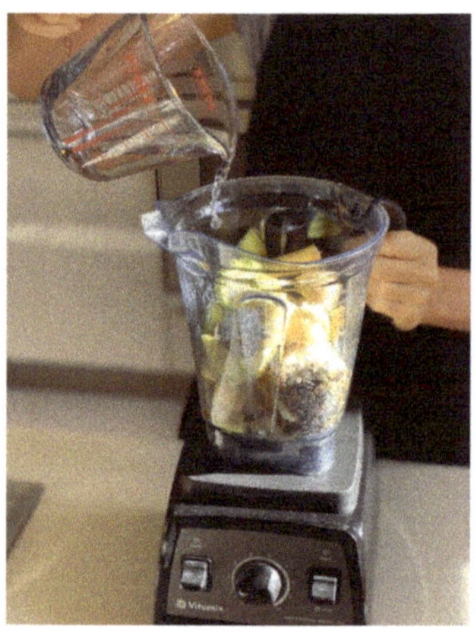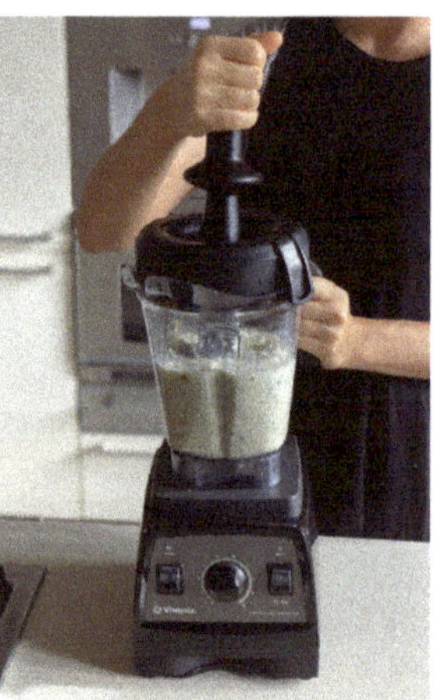

Spread the blended cracker mix evenly on the 14-inch square *Excalibur* dehydrator tray, lined either with a silicon sheet or parchment paper. I very much prefer silicone/Teflex sheets – parchment paper is just an 'okay' temporary solution: you will soon understand why, once you try both. The mixture should be about 3-5mm thick.

I did ask my sweet husband to describe this process in his own words and here is how he put it:

"Empty the freshly blended mix into the center of the silicon sheet on your dehydrating tray. Take a spatula or suitable knife and start spreading the mix from the center out. You're trying to create an even layer of mix covering most of the silicon sheet. Imagine buttering a piece of toast or spreading your favorite jam. Your ambition is to produce an even spread across the silicon sheet about the thickness of a thin crust pizza. Practice makes perfect and you will develop your own technique. There's no right or wrong way. Just YOUR way!"

In general, you want to use 2 to 3 cups of blended cracker mix per 14-inch *Excalibur* dehydrator tray. I recommend over time experimenting with thickness, as really thin and crispy can be a clear preference to some, and thicker, maybe chewy, appeals to others.

The experience of eating crackers of different thicknesses will be very different, despite the fact they are made of the same ingredients.

The last thing to do before placing the trays into the dehydrator and turning the dehydrator on is to score the mix with the butter knife to create lines along which to break up crackers when they have dried. Most of the time I do this step before I place the trays with the blended cracker mix into the dehydrator for the first time – if the cracker mix is thick enough to start with. If the mix is a bit "runny", and you make the lines straight after spreading it on the sheet, they will simply disappear. In that case, wait until the mix dehydrates a little and only then create these lines.

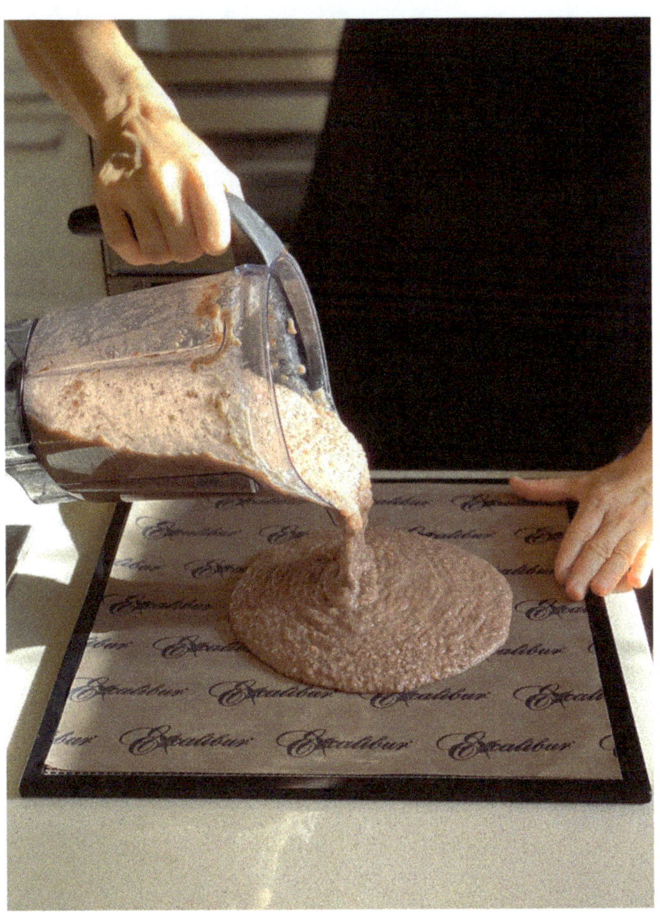

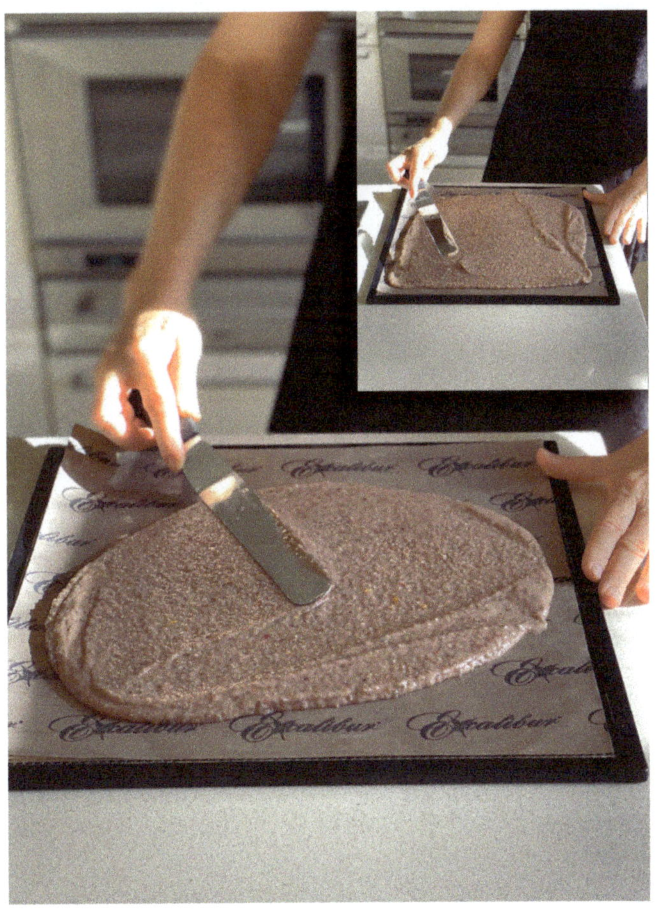

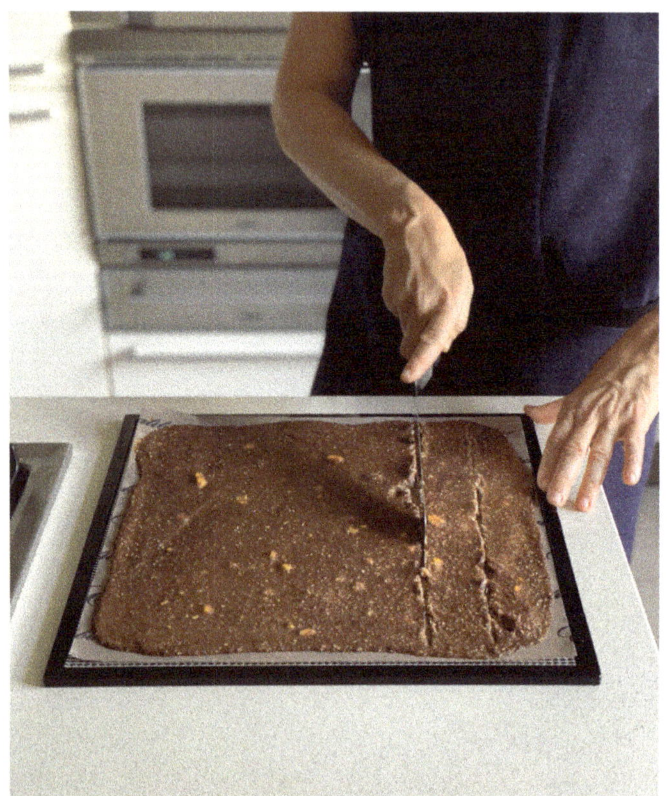 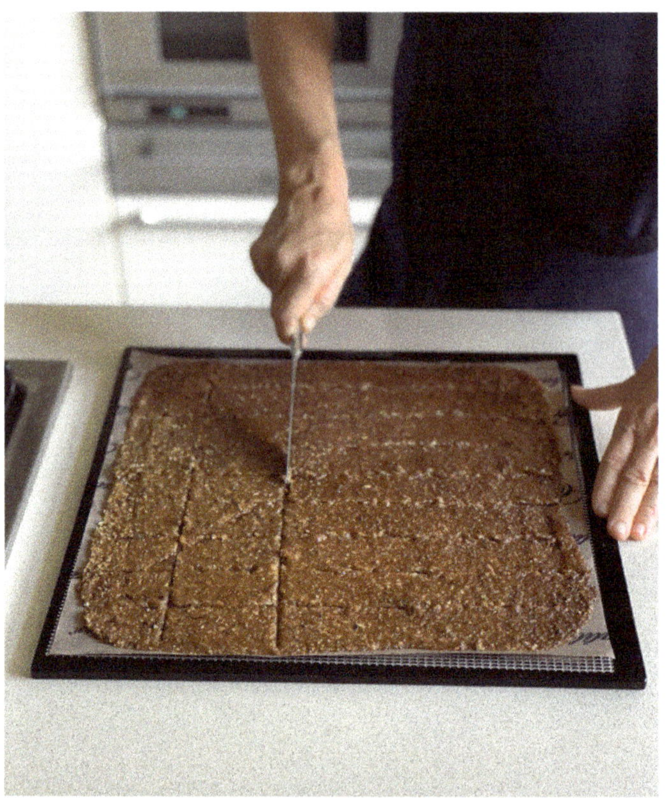

In general, dehydrate for 5 to 6 hours at 104-116°Fahrenheit.

After that, flip your crackers directly onto the mesh tray then peel away the silicon lining or paper. As at this point, they are partially dried, it should be fairly easy to do. You will know if it is good time to do this – once your attempt to peel doesn't tear or break the semi-dry cracker.

The thicker the blended cracker mix consistency at the starting point, the less time it will take to dehydrate.

The thinner the layer you spread, the less time it will take to dehydrate.

The sooner you can peel and flip the drying cracker mix, the faster the final dry consistency develops.

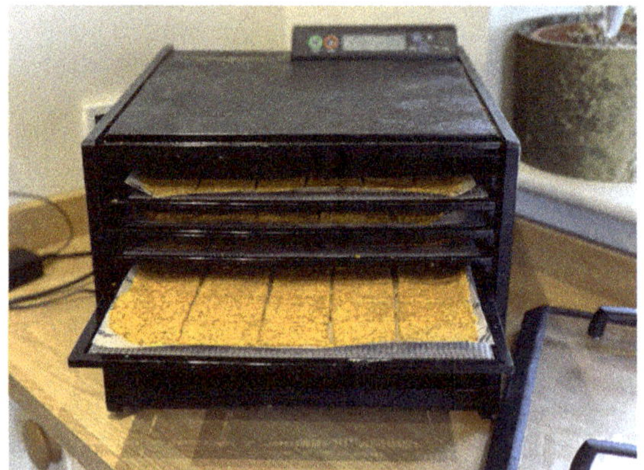

After flipping, dehydrate for another 3-4 hours or until completely dried and crispy. Then remove from the trays and bend along the score lines to break into desired and marked slices/squares/triangles.

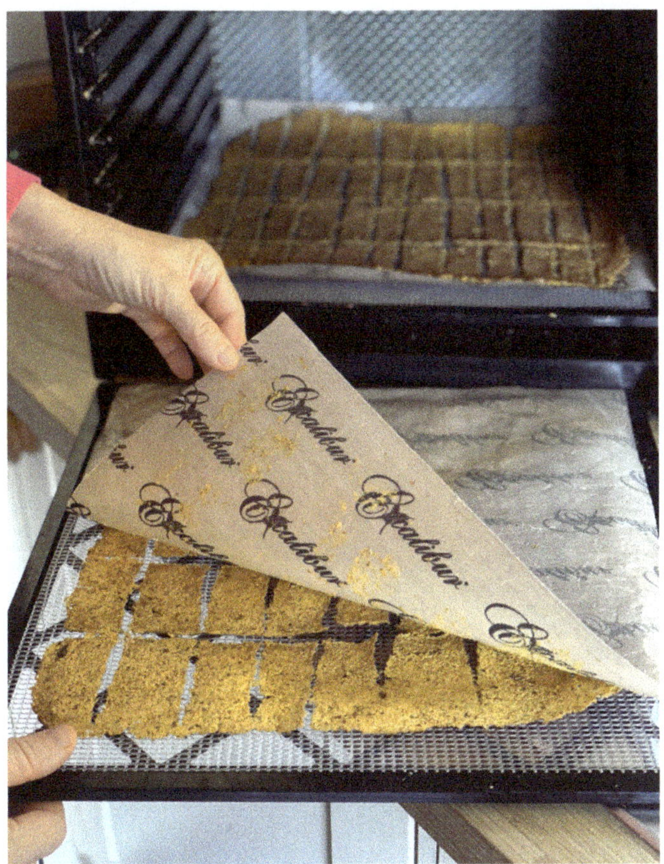

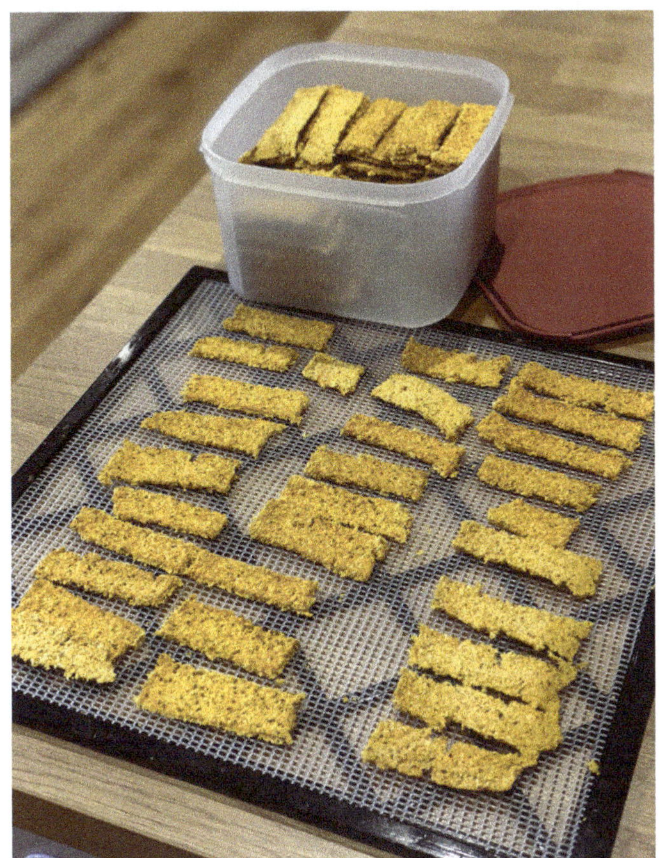

Sometimes you will find that the crackers are already separated completely while dehydrating, so no bending and breaking is required. (Especially if you scored the spread mixture well and the consistency of it was thick from the very start.)

The only thing left to do is stack them into containers and store them nicely.

To make your crackers less crispy, dehydrate for a shorter time. If you feel you left them in the dehydrator for too long simply leave the box with crackers open for a while, they will become softer, absorbing humidity from the outside air.

The best way (when you're only just starting the adventure of 'crackering') to see if the crackers are dry enough is to come to check up on them once in a while. Remove small crackers from the dehydrator, wait until they cool down either on an open site or after being placed in the fridge for 2 minutes (as warm crackers straight from the dehydrator are bendier and softer than the final product will be at room temperature) and then decide if they are ready and done.

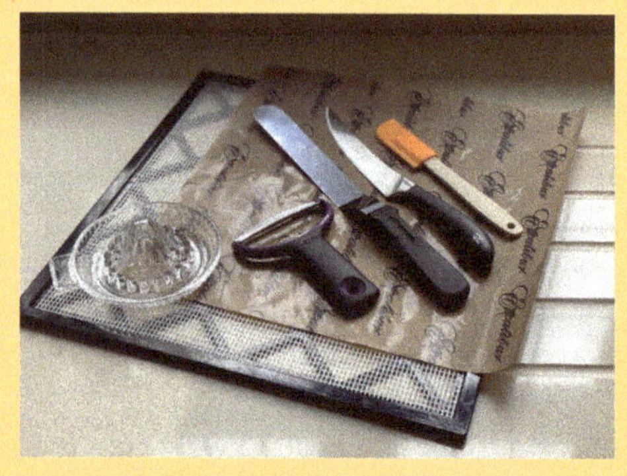
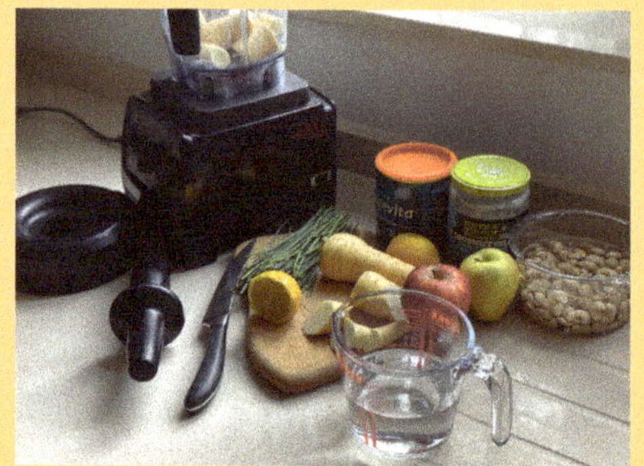
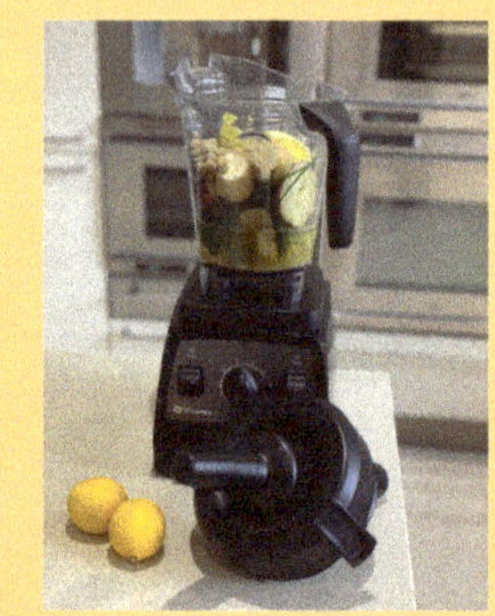
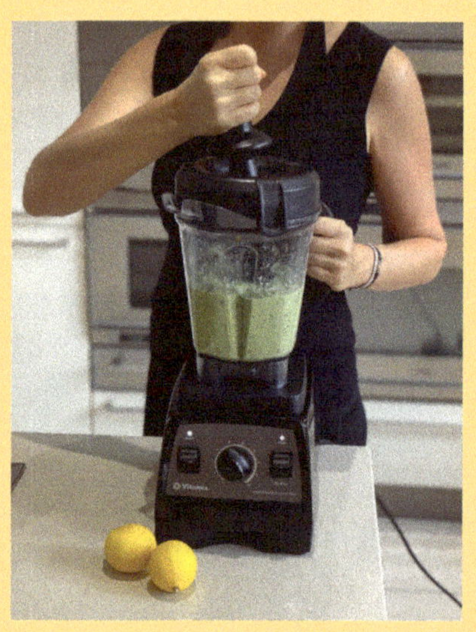
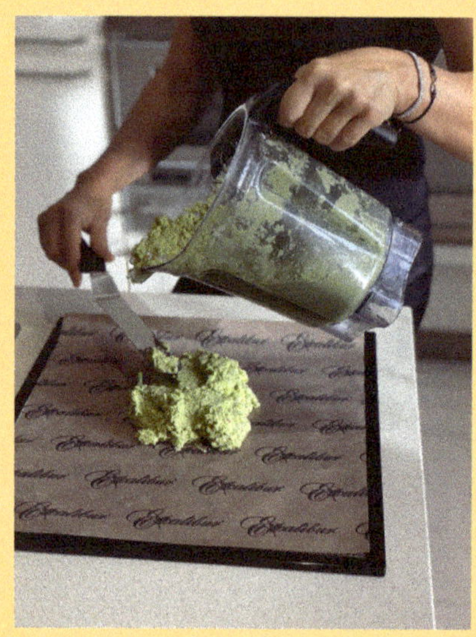
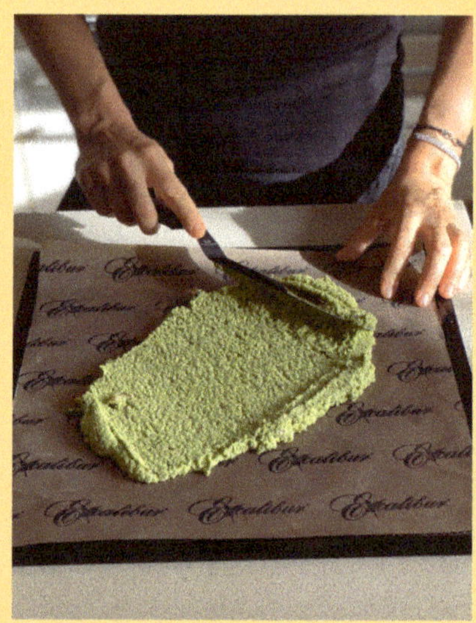
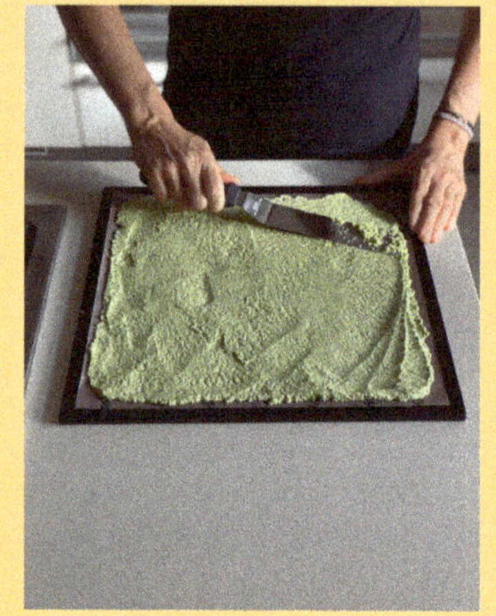
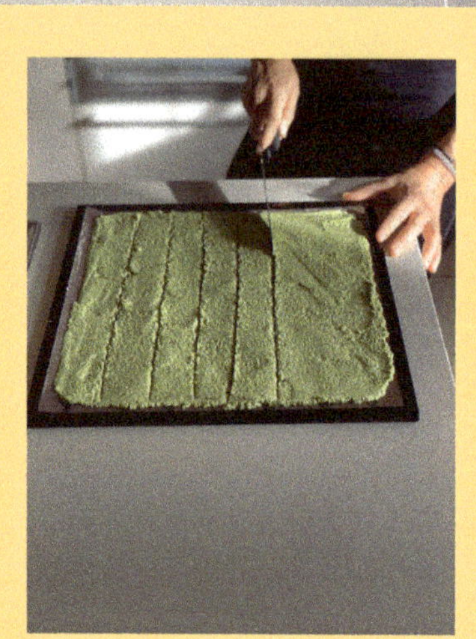
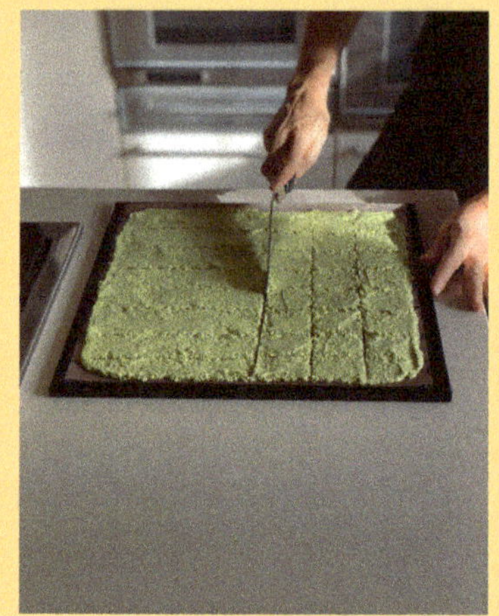

The universal METHOD

Spread the blended cracker mix evenly onto the Teflex sheets lining the dehydrator trays. Once spread evenly (think 'thin pizza crust') try scoring the mixture into slices/squares/triangles, or any other shape you want, with the side of a spatula or blunt knife. If the consistency is too runny for the scoring to take – dehydrate it for a further couple of hours and score it once the cracker mix, now drier, has thickened. Dry at 113 degrees F (45 degrees C) for approx. 5 hours. Check your crackers, flip them and if possible peel them off the sheets. Peeling the crackers from the sheets and leaving them to dry directly on the bare mesh of a dehydrator tray speeds up the process – hence I try to peel the cracker mixture from the sheets as soon as practically possible. Dehydrate for 4-5 hours more. Recheck the crackers and, if crispy-dry, store them in airtight boxes after a brief cooling down. If drying for a little longer is needed, you know what to do.

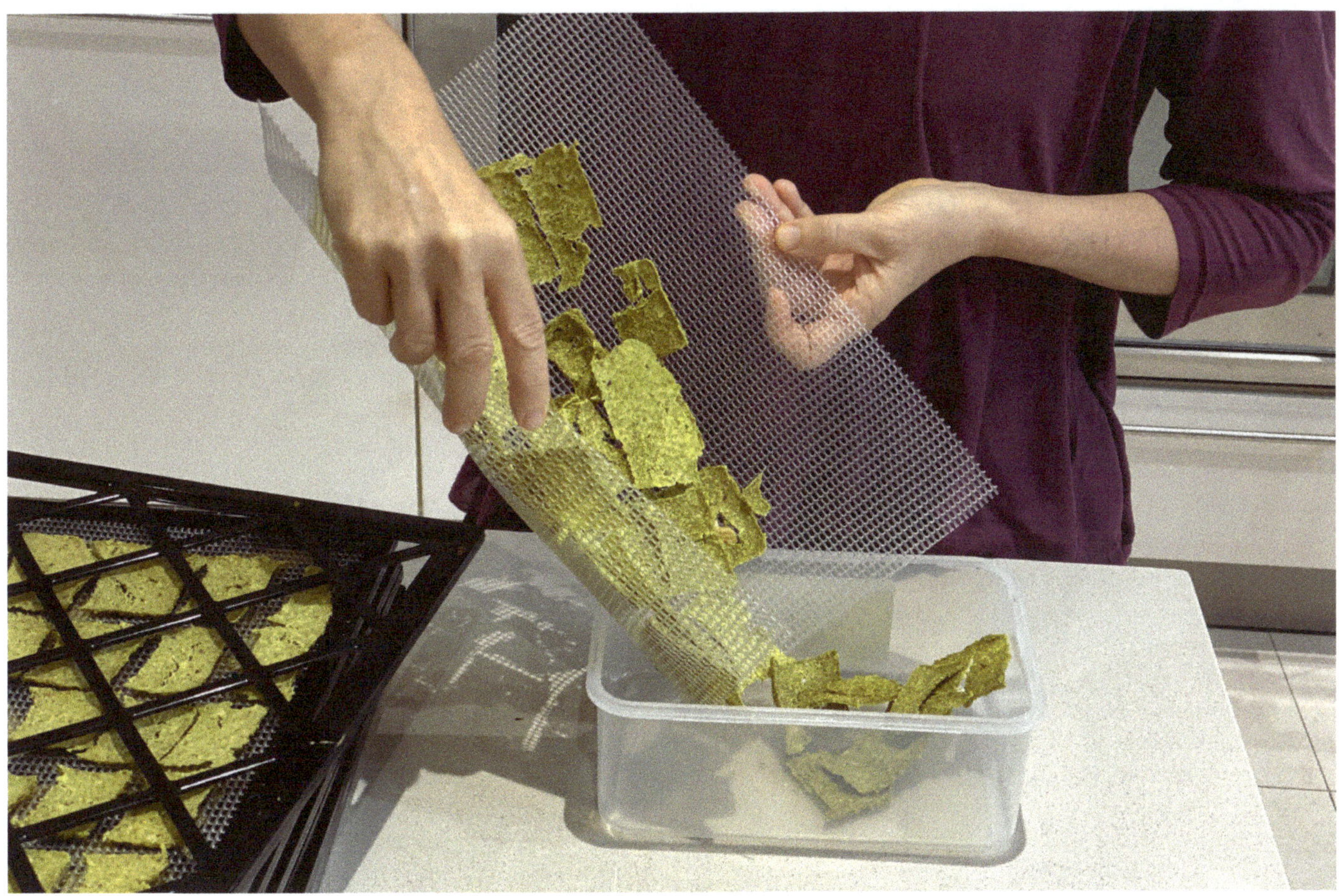

The Perfect Cracker

The PERFECT CRACKER is the ONE YOU (and your nearest and dearest) LOVE! One way to make those successfully is to take my suggested recipes and tweak them into something you and your taste buds absolutely agree with. Experiment!

- For example, you can modify the outcome by amending the ratio of ingredients I mentioned in the recipe, adding fruits/vegetables mentioned as 'optional' in some of the recipes, or simply by adding totally new fruits/veg you feel would be a good fit. You can also skip some of the ingredients I list if they don't feel right for you and your palate. Try a different type of seed or nut than the ones I use in a particular recipe. Add some seeds, try combinations. Get inspired on page number 15… and add some extra goodies and spices (thyme, rosemary, oregano, ginger, cinnamon, cumin, chili, turmeric, nutmeg, cardamom, mustard, garlic, curry powder) for a new twist to your recipe. Doing this, your crackers may even become more healing!

- For fruity recipes, I like to add some lemon or lime juice for an extra zesty kick. For an even tangier result, use some rhubarb or baobab fruit.

- If you really have a sweet tooth and are in the mood for a very sweet cracker you can add a handful of dried dates, honey, stevia leaves, agave syrup, or other natural sweeteners. Very ripe bananas or mangos do the job for me. (I would suggest first trying the recipe without the natural sweeteners, fruits as well veggies have sweetness of their own. You may be surprised by how sweet carrots, red onions, parsnips, beetroot, pumpkin, etc can be.)

- A very small amount of vanilla extract or vanilla bean added to fruity recipes could be THE magic ingredient – rounding out the taste to bring out the creaminess and the balancing sweetness. For the 'luxury upgrade' try adding vanilla to peach, apricot, pear, sweet melon, pineapple, and mango-based crackers.

- You can turn any fruity cracker recipe into one with a caramel 'feel' by adding maca powder.

- Turn any fruity cracker recipe into one with a chocolatey feel by adding cocoa powder, cacao nibs, cacao beans, or carob.

- I feel that adding a couple of pineapple hearts into any fruity cracker recipe enhances the "crispy crunchiness" due to its high fibre content (pineapple contains both soluble and insoluble fibres).

- For playful visual effects and maybe as a novelty for your kids or guests, slice some fruits or vegetables very finely, and place them on top of the cracker BEFORE drying. The way they will look after drying is a surprise! You can create shapes, faces, animals, flowers by positioning bits of different fruits or veggies in the spread cracker mix before drying. Try to sprinkle the whole seeds, finely chopped nuts, or finely chopped onions, chives, olives, sun-dried tomatoes, and press gently into the blended cracker mix before drying.

- Dehydrate for a shorter or longer time than the original recipe suggests.

- Experiment with different thicknesses of the mixture when it's spread out.

- Ingredients you might want to 'see' in the cracker: berries, pieces of olives, tomato, raisins, figs, etc. Add them to the blender almost at the end of the blending process for a very brief last spin, once every other ingredient is blended quite smoothly.

- Try to vary the total time of blending for different final overall textures. What I do sometimes, especially when testing new combos, is blend all the ingredients just to a certain level of smoothness (or un-smoothness) and then remove a portion of the blended mass to spread on the first dehydrator sheet. Continue blending the rest of the cracker mix in the blender for a couple more spins/moments. Stop the blender, take and spread another sample on the second dehydrator sheet. Continue blending what's left over, possibly with a little bit of water added if the blender jug gets more than half empty, until the ingredients become smoother than smooth. I like this level of smoothness for my fruit leathers. See what you think! It is nice to spread an extra thin layer – try and you will see why… Once all these different textured crackers are dried and crispy – ask your kids to tell you which variation is their favorite. These crackers are all the same ingredients in the exact same ratio, but the experience of nibbling on them may differ a lot.

- If you're hungry for savory crackers which are saltier, instead of adding salt you can try adding different types of SEAWEEDS (I prefer to call them SEA VEGETABLES) to amplify your daily intake of antioxidants, iodine, minerals, even vitamin B12. Just be extra careful about from where they have been sourced!

- As I like dark chocolate (the darker the better) I occasionally drizzle melted dark chocolate over dried ready-to-eat crunchy crackers. They look beautiful and taste even better.

- If you or your kids use, or their taste buds really like, some sort of squash (also called cordial or non-alcoholic concentrated sirup) – you could add a hint of it to your fruit cracker mix, as your naughty way to 'help' them to like and give a thumbs up to your first crackering outcome. I personally would not do this- as I prefer pure fully natural flavours. But having an open mind, I decided to share this trick with you anyway. Another way to 'intensify' the fruity flavor in some recipes is to add some sort of dried fruit as an optional addition to the ingredients listed. If I ever do this, it is only in rare cases where I (for some unfortunate reasons) end up with fruit on my hands which didn't ripen totally and I opted not to waste it, but to use it in crackers.

- As the seasons change so may our cravings. You may want to rotate your recipes. To remember which recipe really was a success and made those tasting them ask for more I suggest taking notes during the process. Another easy way is to take a picture of the ingredients piled on your kitchen counter before you proceed to blend them. Store the images with a little text commenting on what was nice about this particular batch, what you would make differently next time, etc, etc. If you feel like it — let me know how it goes and share your cracker story on my Instagram.

STORING

How long do dehydrated foods last? Properly dehydrated, conditioned, and stored dehydrated goodies could last years...

Dry food should be dry enough to prevent microbial growth and subsequent spoilage.

The conditioning of dried goods is a process used to evenly distribute the minimal residual moisture throughout all pieces in the container they are stored in. This reduces the chance of spoilage, especially from mold. This is all theory... For the purposes of this book, I will not go into more details.

What I want to explain is the optimal storage for crackers, and tips on how I do it.

What can sometimes happen to fruit left out too long on your kitchen counter? Especially in warmer weather? Mold. Yes, mold...

Mold is basically bacteria growing and multiplying in favorable external conditions: warmth + humidity + oxygen supply. We obviously don't want mold growing in our crackers. That would mean risking ruining and losing the whole batch, wasting the time and ingredients that went into them and, even worse, tummy ache or food poisoning.

To be on the safe side, I store my crackers in the fridge as often as I can.

Low temperatures significantly lower the chance of bacteria multiplying and prospering. The freezer is another good option if you feel you will not consume them all in the near future.

If I have crackers that are very dry, sometimes I do feel confident enough to leave them on the kitchen counter or cupboard.

What Containers to Use?

In general, airtight containers are what is needed for storing dehydrated foods.

All containers should be cleaned: soap and hot water should be enough, a hot cycle in the dishwasher is even better. What I sometimes do is rinse the container and lid with boiling water. Before placing crackers inside, the containers must be totally dry. Make sure the container and lid don't have knicks and cracks and, if there is any sealing around the lid, that this is not damaged and is placed/snapped on properly.

Option 1

Canning and Mason Jars

You can reuse them again and again. They can also be vacuumed sealed to help extend the life of your crackers. (Remember- that bacteria need oxygen for their life cycle, so if there's little or no oxygen then there's less chance it will grow...)

That said, glass jars, however healthy compared to plastic containers they may be, haven't so far proved to be the best option for me – as time and time again I experience they are not airtight enough meaning that crackers lose their 'crispiness' in a few days if stored in them. I sincerely wanted them to be my #1 choice, as I prefer to minimize contact with plastic as much as possible with the food I eat. It is still a work in progress, and I keep my eyes peeled wherever I travel to find the PERFECT AIRTIGHT GLASS CONTAINERS!! (If you have tips for me, please share them on Instagram Margo.23blossom. I will be grateful.)

Finding the perfect airtight glass container will be great for this planet too...

Option 2

This is where I am at now. I have a bunch of Tupperware containers which keep my crackers totally dry and crispy for a very long time (I mean weeks.) The only thing to be careful with is closing the lid properly each time after snacking.

Option 3

Especially good if you want to store your thicker crackers in the freezer. Be careful though: crackers can be sharp and pointy, they can puncture the plastic and ruin your hard work by allowing air to get in, through even the smallest of the puncture holes... The solution to this is either to get thicker plastic bags or/and wrap the dried crackers in parchment paper before inserting them into a vacuum seal bag for sealing. This helps protect the bags from punctures.

Option 4

These are the ones I keep my crackers in for short trips and travels. For smaller quantities of crackers to take on a walk with your little one, they easily fit into your handbag and still remain crispy if left for a few days.

Once again I am still looking for the perfect brand, so I can recommend it to you too one day.

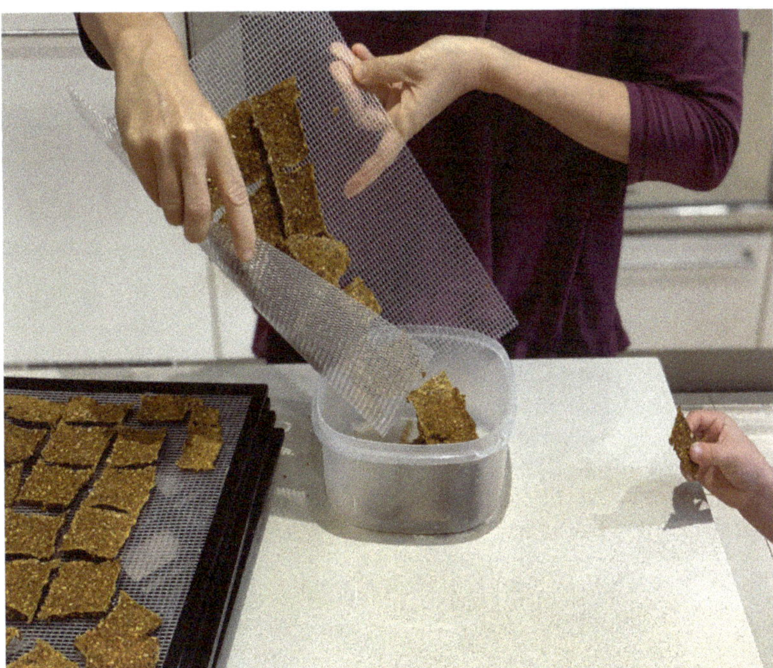

Last Tip

LABEL YOUR containers and jars. Once you have more than a few batches, this will become helpful. You will see what I mean! Some of them may look quite similar!

Dehydrating DOs and DON'Ts

These little snippets of information are in no particular order, I just thought them worthwhile mentioning:

- Ensure that you occasionally clean your dehydrator with tepid water. Clean the base of the dehydrator because food tends to collect at this part.

- Never leave your dehydrator Teflex sheets stacked wet. Mold will take over.

- Keep the dehydrator and cable far away and safe from small kids.

- As mentioned before, make sure the fan of the dehydrator is allowed free airflow. Don't place it too close to the wall, other surfaces, or in small cupboards. Do not cover the dehydrator while using it.

- Use a good-quality dehydrator that circulates the heated air evenly and maintains a consistent temperature. Otherwise, you run the risk of bad bacteria or mold growth developing and, possibly, unevenly dehydrated crackers.

- If you're dehydrating overnight using a timer – make sure you set the timer for long enough to allow sufficient time for dehydrating (the dehydrating time will of course vary depending on the natural levels of moisture, sugar and the type of dehydrator). Over time and with more experience (and cracker trays successfully made) you will be able to estimate the dehydrating time with more accuracy. At the beginning, set the dehydrator for longer rather than shorter. The reason for this is the same as the one above, to avoid the bacteria growing while the crackers are 'humid'.

- Make your blended cracker mix wet but not too runny. Dehydrating will take much less time.

- Crackers on trays sitting closest to the the dehydrator fan will dry more quickly than the rest. Rotating drying trays every few hours can alleviate this.

- Try to score the cracker mixture spread on Teflex sheets as soon as possible before or while dehydrating. This will shorten the time needed for thorough dehydrating. The same goes for flipping and peeling off the Teflex sheets. Crackers placed on bare dehydrator tray meshes dry much faster.

- Dry the crackers thoroughly and then allow them to cool to room temperature before enclosing them in an airtight container. Dried items taken directly out of a dehydrator can 'sweat' even though their moisture content is low, so allowing a couple of minutes of cooling off before sealing them in a container will ensure that moisture is not trapped inside.

- When storing, remember to label the containers with the name of the crackers (main flavor/ingredient) and possibly the date when you made them.

- Close the box where the crackers are stored properly, otherwise they will get humid quite quickly (as they absorb water content from the atmosphere). Humid crackers are chewier, less crispy and less crunchy. If this happens, the solution is simple, fast, and easy. Place them in the dehydrator on the bare tray mesh to re-dehydrate for a couple of hours back to their original perfection.

- If possible, store your crackers in the fridge or freezer rather than at room temperature. The main reasons for this are: to extend the shelve life, to limit the possibility of bacteria and mold growth, and to improve the crunch experience. (Eating crackers chilled, straight from the fridge will be a crispier experience as the fat contained within will be in solid state.)

- Try to avoid dehydrating garlic and onion spiced crackers together with sweet treats at the same time. You can guess why…

- Remember that your seasonings will be twice as strong after drying.

- Do not attempt to dry your crackers in a microwave.

- Last but not least, not directly related to dehydrating but still worth mentioning, do not bin any of the overripe fruit, little 'tired' veggies from your fridge, and of course your pulp from the juicing. If you cannot use them right now - freeze them for future crackering.

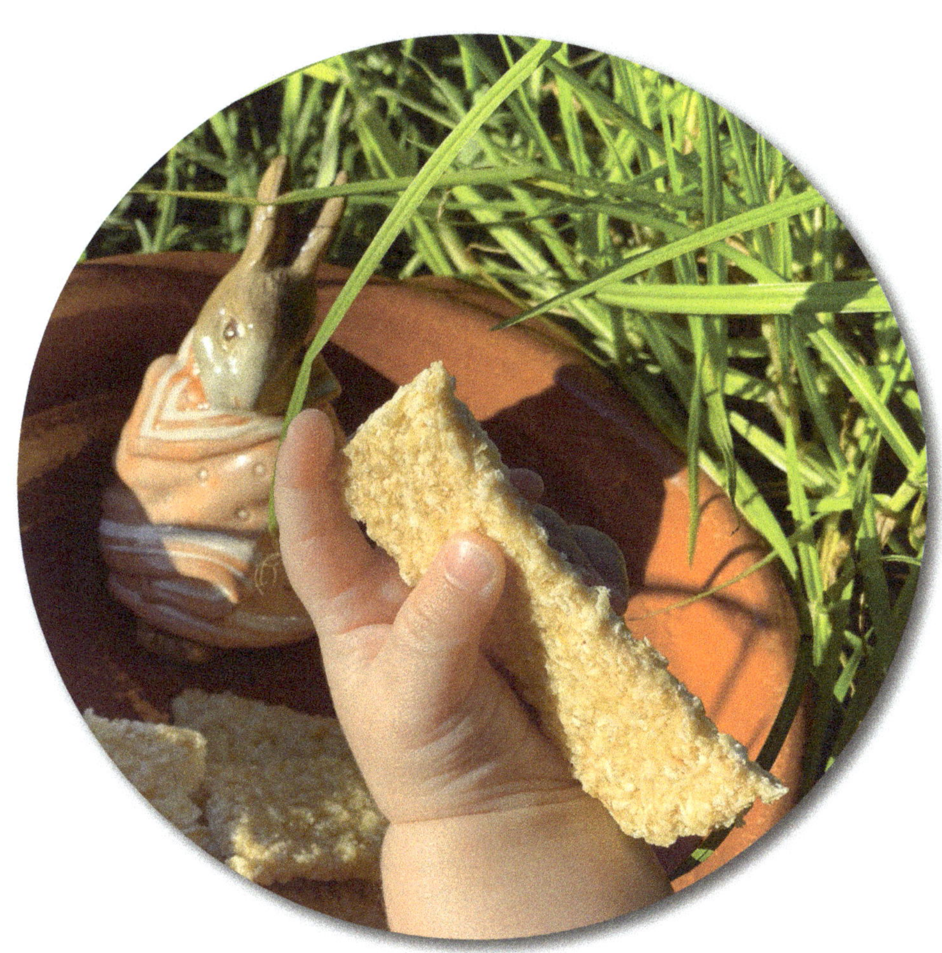

Allergies. A few words...

(Before proceeding to the recipes which is where all the fun will begin, let's get the 'A' word out of the way!)

How to Spot an Allergy

After introducing nuts (or seeds, as sometimes these are produced/packaged around nuts), or fruits & veggies your child has never had before, you should check for the following signs of allergies:

Rashes

Vomiting

Wheezing

Runny nose

Swelling of lips and face

Itchy eyes

If you spot these allergy indications, it is recommended to reach out to your pediatrician (or if in the UK you can use the NHS 111 for advice) without delay! Use emergency services (UK 999, USA 911, Europe 112) if the reaction is severe.

It seems nowadays human bodies may develop allergies to some fruits and veggies too. Quite a wild world we live in... I would say be very vigilant; especially if it is the first time you are introducing some new food to your child regardless of what it is. It is not the beautiful fruit, vegetable, seed, or nut which hurts the human body and should be called the 'bad guy'...

There is a story (and history) behind each and every case. I personally believe your child's body is influenced and, in a way, conditioned for potential future allergies from the very start of its development. That means foods, drinks, cosmetics, even the air the mother is breathing, can all play a role. The next stage of this conditioning happens in the very first few months of the baby's life – especially if being breastfed – by everything the breastfeeding mother eats, drinks, as well applies to her skin.

Big no-no's are artificial sweeteners, processed foods, drinks, and meals containing food colorants and preservatives, chemically treated or inorganically grown fruits and veggies... the list can be long.

Last, I must mention one more potential reason for allergies so you can hopefully avoid it. And that is premature and rushed weaning: introducing food groups and processed foods to the baby's diet too early and/or too fast. If you have a small baby who is about to be introduced to solid food for the first time, please DO NOT RUSH the weaning! Taking it slowly is the key! Introducing new foods gradually and as mono-meals at the very beginning is a safe way to proceed. The tiny body and its systems and organs is still developing. It is not ready for overload. The lining of the intestinal tract is delicate and its permeability is not yet where it needs to be to safely handle complex meal combos, food groups such as complex proteins, processed foods with additives etc. before 7-8 months of age. The same goes for the baby's kidneys. It is all a work in progress especially in the first year. Wean slowly, with caution and patience. Not introducing new food groups way too early is a great way to prevent potential allergies in the future. For more details and my views on how to wean your baby safely, check my book *Go Wild*.

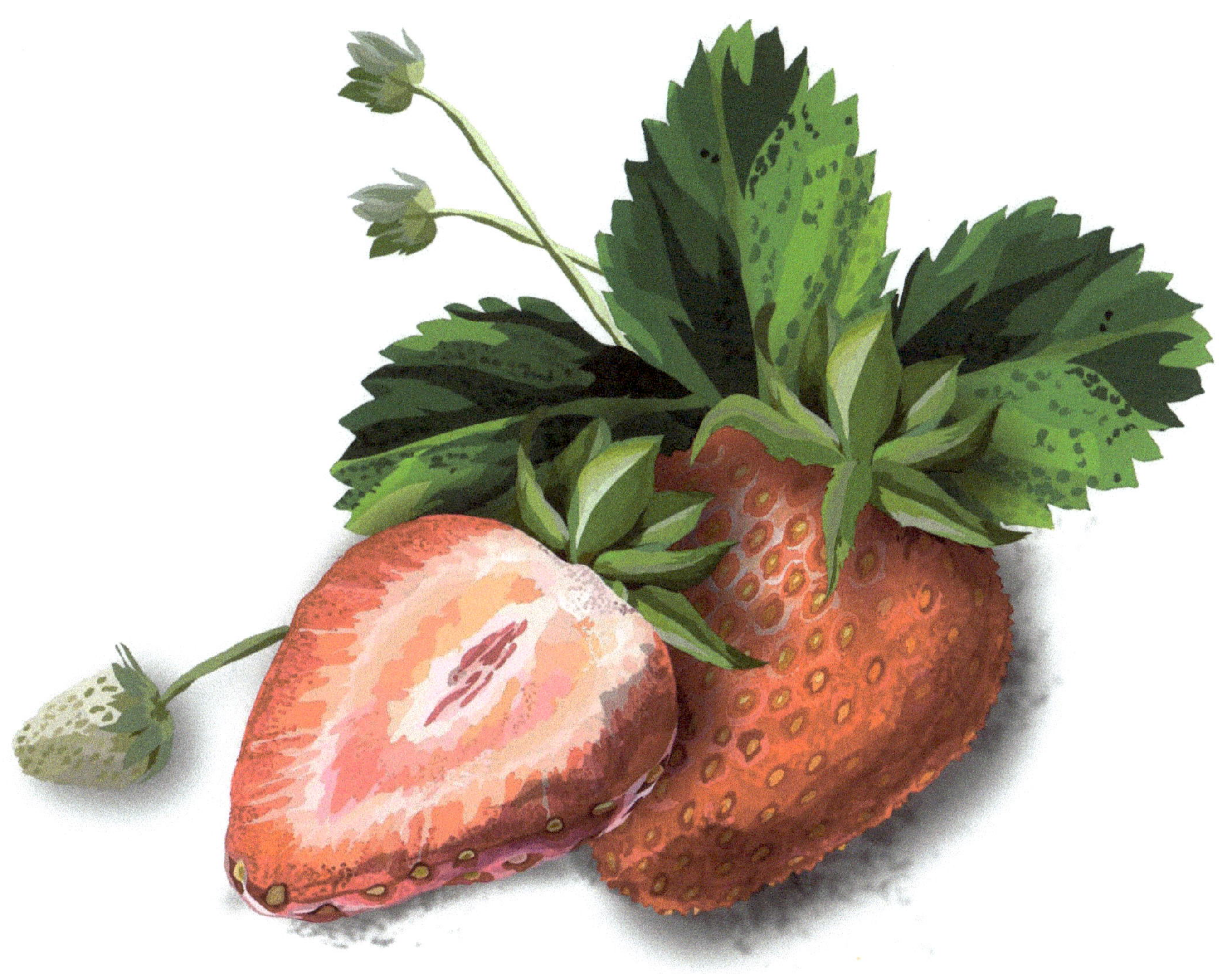

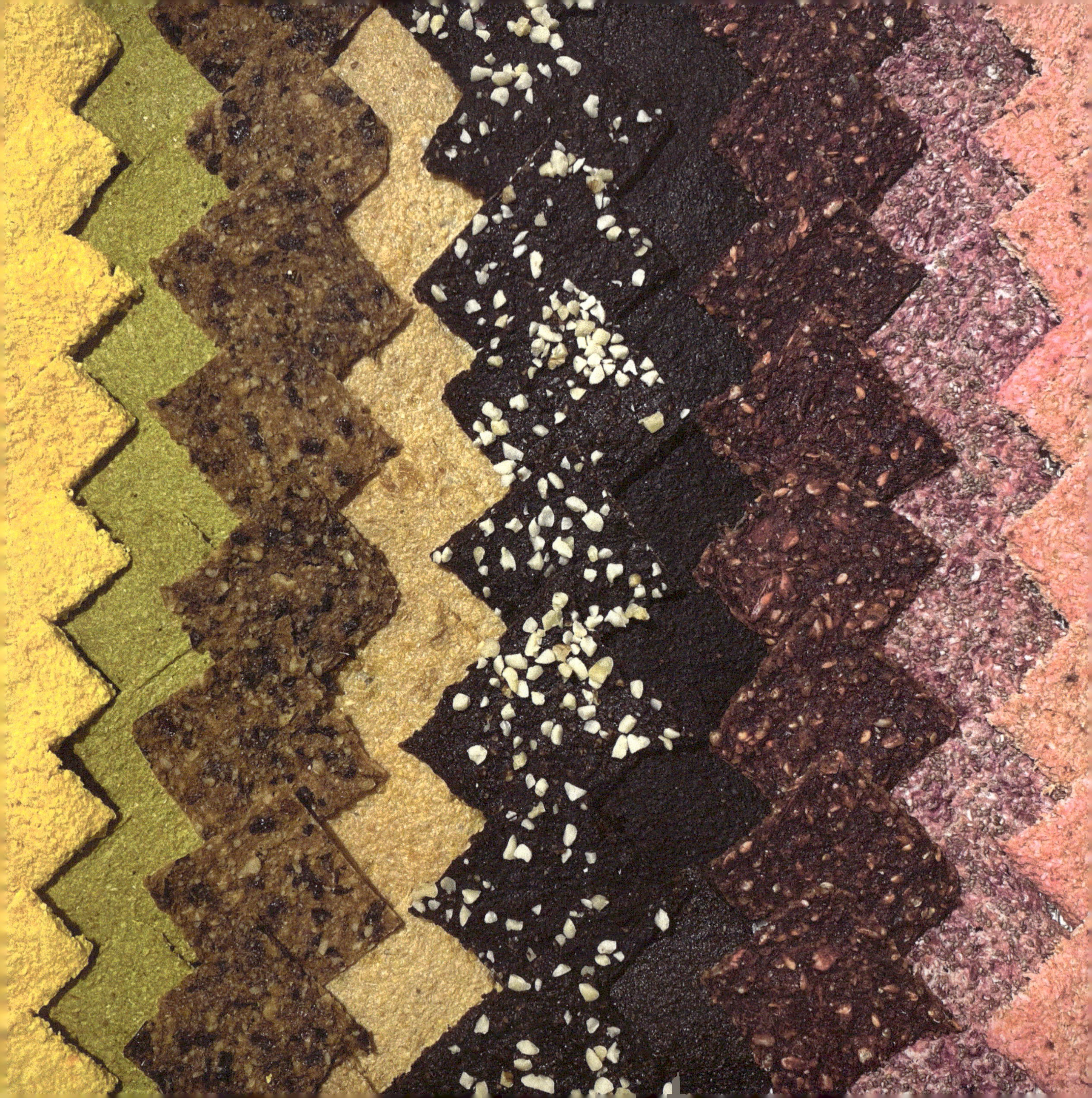

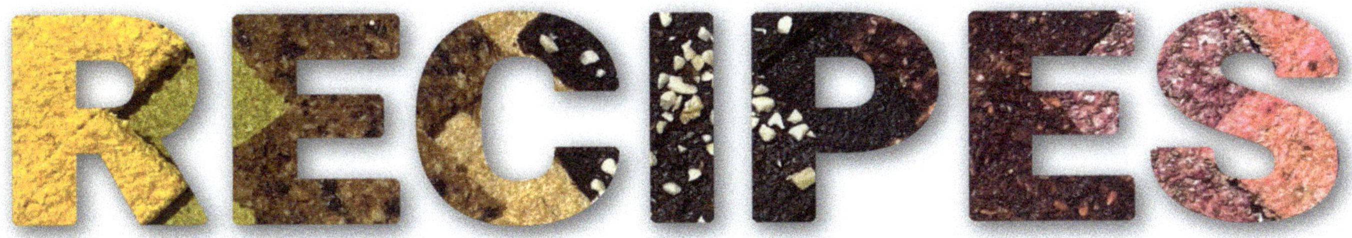

Radiant RASPBERRY

Did you ever walk in the forest where wild raspberries grow? It feels magical. Especially if you happen to be hungry… For berries…

I treasure memories like that.

As with all berries, raspberries are rich in vitamin C, containing vitamin B1, B2, B3, B5, B6, folate, vitamin E, vitamin K and an array of minerals such as manganese, calcium, iron, magnesium, phosphorus, potassium, zinc. So yes, definitely good for you and your little ones.

Do you favor the raspberry flavor?

If yes, here is the list of ingredients for quick, smart, raspberry crackers.

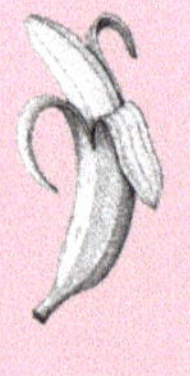

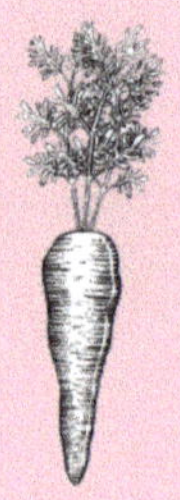

Ingredients:

1 kg berries (or as many as you can get)

3 ripe bananas

2 carrots

2 parsnips

1 level tablespoon of coconut oil

Bag of mixed raw seeds (300g)

Optional:

*To make this recipe 'chocolatey' raspberry, add **cocoa powder or nibs.***

Once again – in case you were wondering – it is not hard to grow your own. Raspberries are vigorous and can even be locally invasive. They propagate using basal shoots – extended underground shoots that develop roots and individual plants – so they can take over your garden if left unattended. I'm speaking here from my own experience! Raspberries are often propagated using cuttings and will root readily in moist soil conditions. You should give it a try!

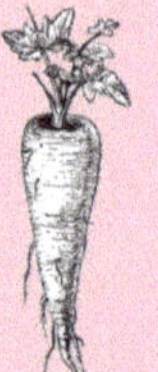

Process

Cut the cleaned carrots and parsnips into 2-3 cm pieces (this will make the blending easier). Place them in the blender together with coconut oil, seeds, bananas, berries and start blending. If necessary add some warm water. I always use the tamper while blending my cracker mix, as it helps the process and keeps the blender safe. Blend until the texture of the cracker mix looks good to you.

Spread the blended cracker mix evenly on the Teflex sheet placed on the dehydrator tray. Once spread evenly (think thin pizza crust thickness) try to score the mixture with the side of the spatula or blunt knife into slices or squares. If the consistency of the mix is still too runny, dehydrate it for a couple of hours and score it once the mixture has thickened (this means it's drier).

Dry at 113 degrees F (45 degrees C) for approx. 5 hours. Check upon your crackers, flip them and peel off the silicone sheets if possible. Peeling the crackers off silicone sheets and leaving them on a bare dehydrator tray mesh makes drying much faster… hence I try to peel the blended cracker mix from silicone sheets as soon as it's possible.

Dehydrate for 4-5 hours more.

Check upon crackers again and, if crispy dry, store in airtight boxes after a brief cooling down.

If drying for a little longer is needed, you know what to do.

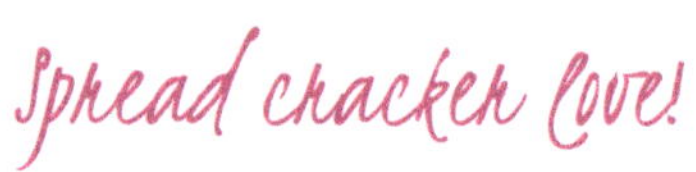

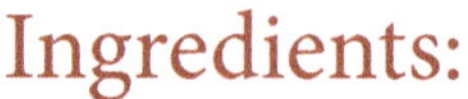

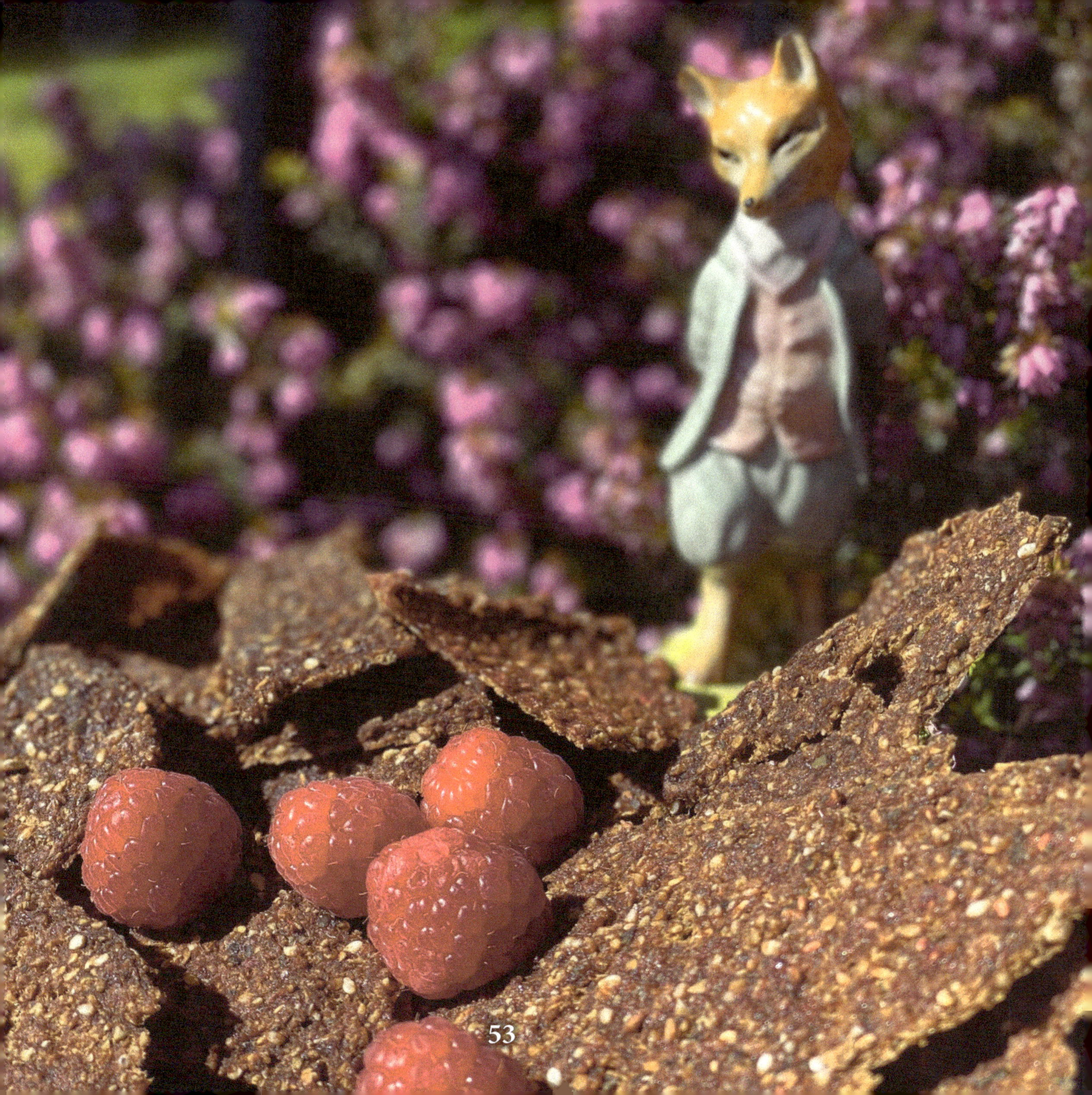

2

Perfect PINEAPPLE and COCONUT

Does the thought of this delicious combo bring back yummy memories from your sunny holiday in the Caribbean or southeast Asia? Pineapple, or the ananas plant, which Columbus brought back to Spain from his Latin American voyage (he called it "Pine of the Indians" by the way) contains loads of manganese, vitamin C, and fiber. It also contains antioxidants, vitamin B, copper, thiamine, folate, potassium magnesium, riboflavin, iron, as well as phytochemicals and enzymes aiding digestion and having an anti-inflammatory effect on the human body. Put it this way: Pineapples are really good for us!

In our household, we eat pineapples on a daily basis. The middle part or the core (I like to call it the heart of pineapple) is quite fibrous, hence hard to chew. I treasure and collect all these pineapple hearts and keep them in a freezer in Tupperware containers or ziplock bags, as they add a nice crunchy texture to crackers. (Well – you know – we can still consider them an edible part of the plant and avoid wasting food!)

Having gathered a pile of them – it's time to prepare these mouthwatering crackers.

Ingredients:

1 perfectly ripe pineapple (or 10-15 pineapple hearts)

1 mature coconut

2-3 ripe bananas

1-2 parsnips

Optional:

Carrots/apple, Pumpkin, Hemp seeds, Fruit of baobab powder (adds some lovely "tanginess"), Dash of **lemon/lime juice**

**If the coconuts you are using are "young", how many you may need depends on how much coconut flesh (or 'meat' as some people call it) is developed. You will see what is in them only after you open them. Apply approximately a 1:3 weight ratio of young coconut meat to pineapple. I have to say I personally prefer to use mature coconuts for this recipe. If you can't lay your hands on a whole coconut, improvise and use unsweetened desiccated coconut instead.*

***If you drink young coconuts often, collect the coconut meat and store the stash in the freezer. It can be handy for all sorts of different uses aside from these crackers.*

Process

Peel the pineapple, cut it into smaller pieces, and place it into a blender.

(Alternatively use the pineapple hearts. It helps to cut these into halves before placing them in the blender.) Break the mature coconut and remove the flesh from the shell. *** If you are wondering how to do this without getting your whole kitchen (including walls and ceiling) dirty or hurting yourself with the hammer, here's my inspiring method! I take the mature coconut out in the garden and let it 'fall' on a hard surface such as a patio a couple of times as needed. The impact cracks the nutshell in a couple of places, and if you get lucky, can still keep the white flesh whole and intact without losing the water. With the help of a knife, carefully prise/cut out the pieces of coconut meat from the coconut shell.

Add these coconut pieces to a blender, as well parsnips and a cup of filtered water. (You could use the coconut water from a young coconut instead.)

Blend first to homogenize the hard bits of parsnips, coconut and pineapple hearts a little, before adding the softer ingredients such as banana into the blender.

Blend everything until the cracker mix has the texture you like. I like mine kind of 'grainy 'so that I still see tiny pieces of coconut in the dried crackers.

Continue with the METHOD on pages 40-41

The best cracker in the world!

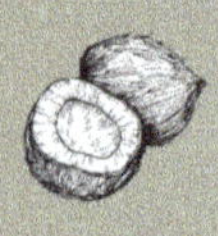

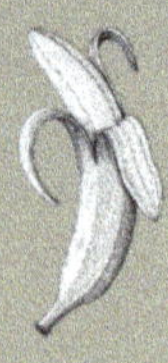

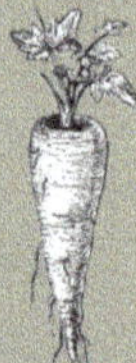

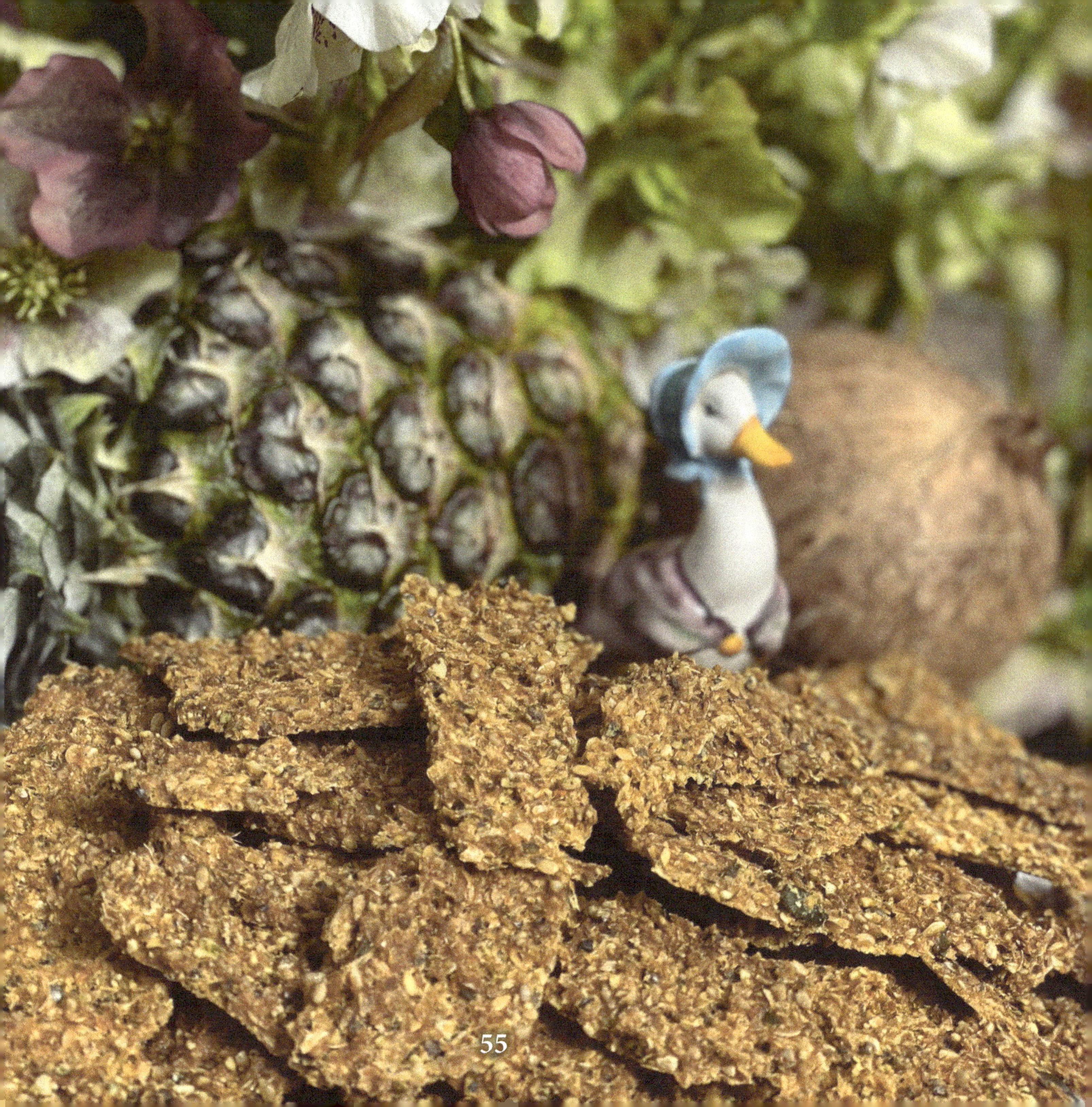

3

Perky PAPAYA and PUMPKIN

Does papaya grow in your climate? Do you have access to this fruit in its fresh and organic state? If you do, this is a nice combo for you to try.

Is the memory of this lovely, sweet, fresh papaya taste still with you from your last holiday breakfast in the luscious tropics and are you craving the recreation of it — but have no fresh papaya within your reach? You can always improvise and use dried papaya. In this case, make sure you soak it for a couple of hours before using it, and remember not to use the soaking water.

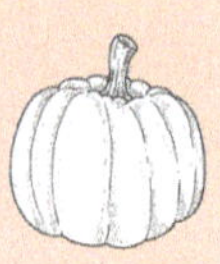

Papayas are fast-growing shade trees and they look really good. Papaya originated in the lowland tropics of South America, but today you find papayas growing everywhere in the tropics and subtropics. It often grows wild, and every tropical food garden has several papaya trees. They grow fast in favorable conditions and bear fruit all year around.

To grow good papayas, you need a frost-free climate, lots of sunlight, lots of water, and very good soil.

If you can supply all of the above you can pretty much stick some papaya seeds in the ground at any time of the year, and six to ten months later they will start fruiting. I could write more about the matter, for example about the fact there are male and female plants, and that you want mostly female plants in your garden, with just a couple of male ones for pollination...

But the recipe awaits…!

Ingredients:

1 big ripe fresh papaya (the bigger the better)

(alternatively use 500g of dried papaya)

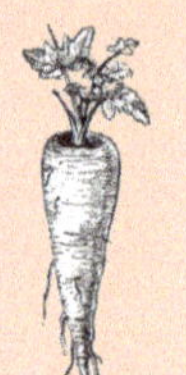

1/2 pumpkin or butternut squash

3 parsnips

1 bag (300g) raw mixed seeds or 300g of yellow flaxseeds

1 level tablespoon of raw coconut oil

Optional:

*Feel free to add some **vanilla pod** (essence)*

1-2 apples

1-2 ripe bananas

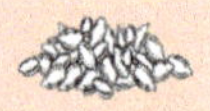

PS: fresh ripe papaya in its original form is one of my favorite first safe baby foods.

Process

Peel papayas, pumpkin, and lemon, removing the seeds.

(I do not use papaya seeds and skin in this recipe. I read somewhere though that these seeds have strong antiparasitic properties, so feel free to test them and let me know how it went if you decide to keep the seeds.)

Blend all the ingredients with up to a cup of filtered water until you are happy with the smoothness of the cracker mix. I am done blending when I still see and recognize some seed bits in the blend.

Spread the blended cracker mix evenly on the Teflex sheet placed on the dehydrator tray. Once spread evenly (think thin pizza crust) try to score the mix with the side of the spatula or blunt knife into slices or squares. If the consistency is still too runny – dehydrate it for a couple more hours and score it once the cracker mix thickens (meaning it's drier). Dry at 113 degrees F (45 degrees C) for approx. 5 hours. Check your crackers, flip them and peel off the sheets if possible. Peeling the crackers off sheets and leaving them on a bare mesh of dehydrator tray makes drying much faster – hence I try to peel the cracker mix from the sheets as soon as it's possible. Dehydrate for 4-5 hours more. Recheck the crackers and, if crispy-dry, store them in airtight boxes after a brief cooling down. If drying for a little longer is needed, you know what to do.

Have a fun cracker day!

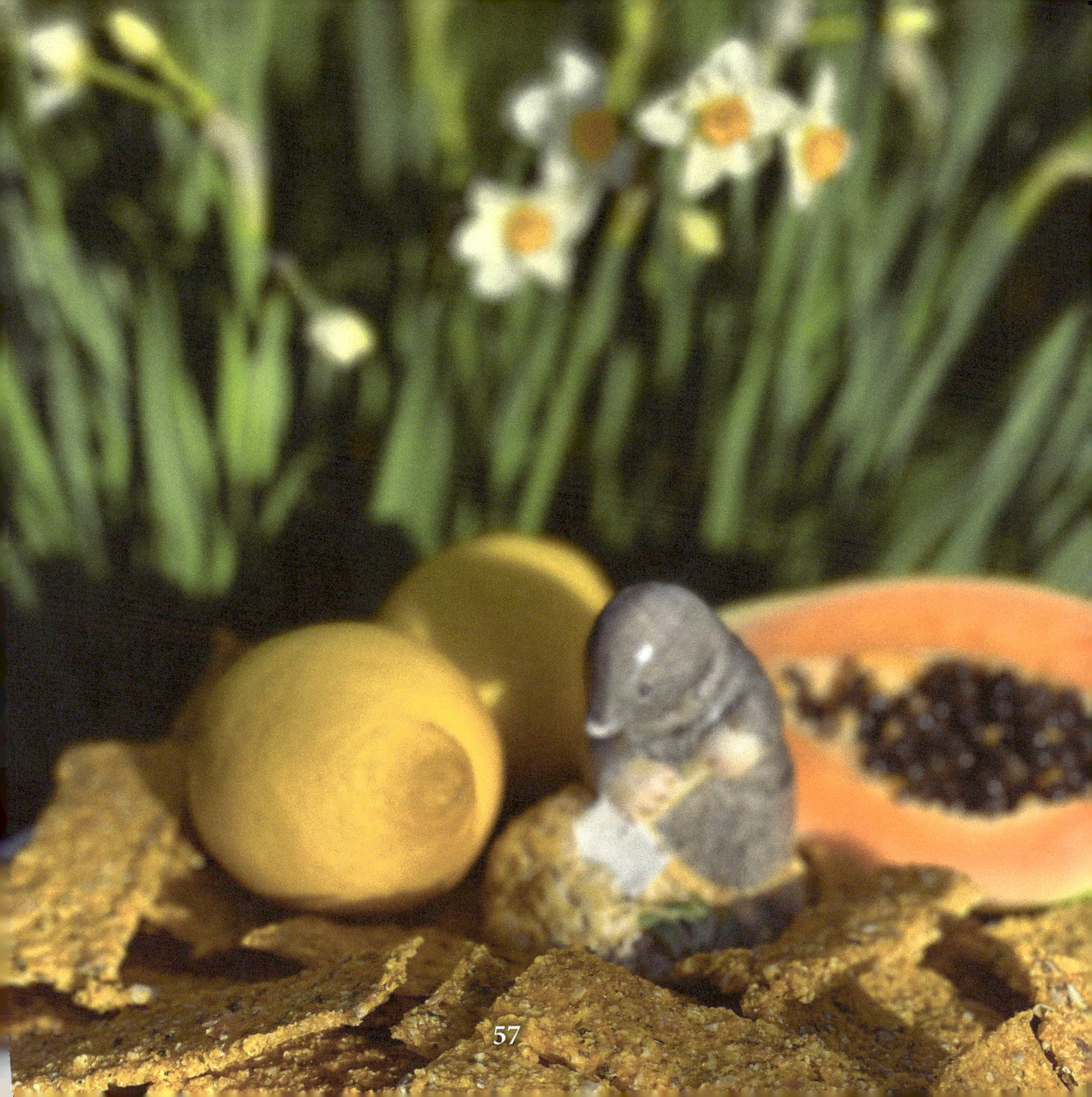

4

Brilliant BEETROOT and CRANBERRY

Did you ever see a harvest of cranberries? These tiny 'tart' fruits contain 4 air pockets hence they float on the water. The sight of cranberry beds ("bogs") filled with water at harvest time (which is usually in October and November in the major cranberry growing regions of the USA) is quite spectacular. Tons of red berries, looking like seas of a RED magic potion, in contrast with blue skies above...

Talking about the impressive shades of red nature gifts us – beetroot is WOW! I looove fresh beetroot juice. With a bit of ginger, and maybe lemon and apple. It is a real treat. If you're juicing beetroot at home, try to use the pulp for this brilliant cracker recipe.

And if you're not a fan of juicing, this recipe can still be a great way to introduce this wonderful healing vibrant vegetable to your kid's diet.

Ingredients:

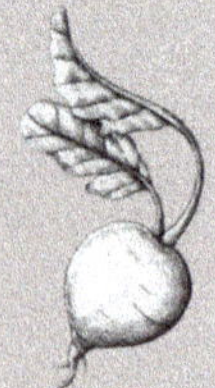

3-5 medium to large beetroots

(or pulp leftovers from juicing)

700 g of fresh cranberries (if can't get fresh, frozen or dried are a fine alternative.) Remember to soak and rinse the dried cranberries, if you opt for using those, before adding them to the blender.

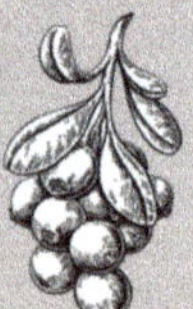

2-3 parsnips

300 g raw mixed seeds

1 level tablespoon of raw coconut oil

As a twist or tweak to this original recipe – feel free to add ripe bananas, apples, or oranges.

Process

Place all the hard ingredients together with coconut oil, seeds and cup of warm water in the blender. Whizz for 2-3 minutes, using the tamper while blending, as it helps the process and keep your blender safe. Add cranberries, and blend until the texture of the cracker mix looks good to you.

Spread the blended cracker mix evenly on the Teflex sheet placed on the dehydrator tray. Once spread evenly (think thin pizza crust) try to score the mix with the side of the spatula or blunt knife into slices or squares. If the consistency is still too runny – dehydrate it for a couple more hours and score it once the cracker mix thickens (meaning it's drier). Dry at 113 degrees F (45 degrees C) for approx. 5 hours. Check your crackers, flip them and peel off the sheets if possible. Peeling the crackers off sheets and leaving them on a bare mesh of dehydrator tray makes drying much faster – hence I try to peel the cracker mix from the sheets as soon as it's possible. Dehydrate for 4-5 hours more. Recheck the crackers and, if crispy-dry, store them in airtight boxes after a brief cooling down. If drying for a little longer is needed, you know what to do.

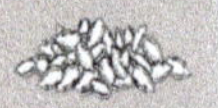

Sit back and bite the cracker!

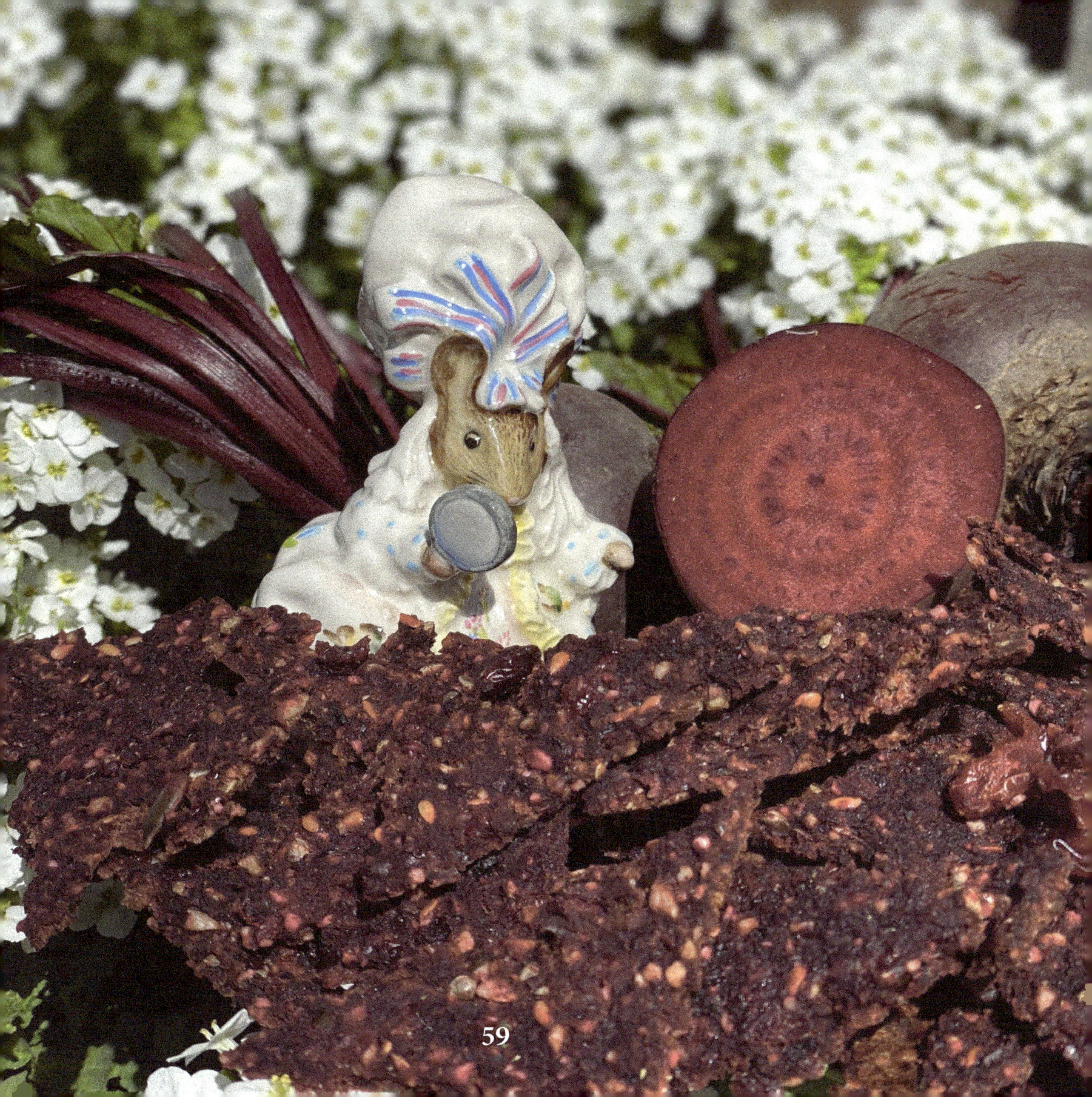

5

Heavenly chocolatey crackers with RAISINS and SPINACH

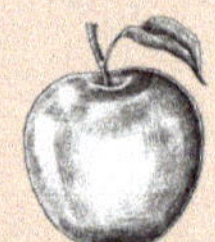

Is it just my observation or do all toddlers like raisins? Do you have a naughty 2 or 3-year-old who doesn't stop moving? Give them a little box of raisins and suddenly they'll sit down, stop talking, and focus on one little dried grape after another filling their mouth, being entertained for a long while.

Let's take advantage of the kids of the world loving the taste of raisins and the chewy texture – and hide a huge amount of greens within this yummy chocolatey treat. Do you like this idea?

Ingredients

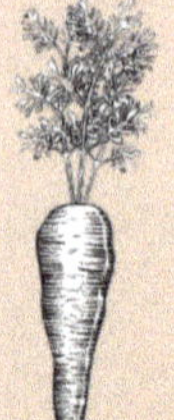

2 apples

3 carrots/parsnips

1-3 ripe bananas

500g of raisins (soak and rinse well before adding)

1 big bag of fresh organic spinach (no one just you will know how big a bunch you managed to sneakily throw in)

1 level tablespoon of raw coconut oil

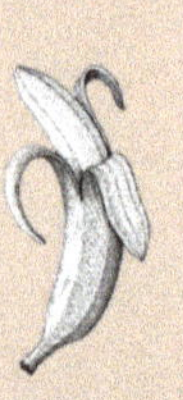

300 g of raw mixed seeds or just one type of seed of your(I opted for sunflower)

Cocoa powder (unsweetened) and/ or raw cocoa nibs for a more crunchy texture. (I used 3 heaped tablespoons)

Process

Place all the ingredients in a blender with a cup of filtered warm water. Blend until you like the structure of the blended mass. I usually leave the raisins out and add them only by the end of blending time. This way some little bits of raisins remain whole and make the experience of tasting your kid's favorite treat in crackers more convincing.

Spread the blended cracker mix evenly on the Teflex sheet placed on the dehydrator tray. Once spread evenly (think thin pizza crust) try to score the mix with the side of the spatula or blunt knife into slices, squares or triangles. If the consistency is still too runny – dehydrate it for a couple more hours and score it once the cracker mix thickens (meaning it's drier). Dry at 113 degrees F (45 degrees C) for approx. 5 hours. Check your crackers, flip them and peel off the sheets if possible. Peeling the crackers off sheets and leaving them on a bare mesh of dehydrator tray makes drying much faster – hence I try to peel the cracker mix from the sheets as soon as it's possible. Dehydrate for 4-5 hours more. Recheck the crackers and, if crispy-dry, store them in airtight boxes after a brief cooling down. If drying for a little longer is needed, you know what to do.

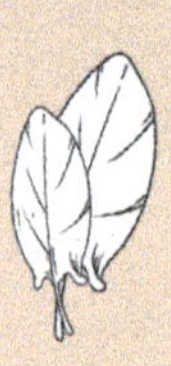

I know how hard it can be to make kids eat green leaves in the form of a salad. In fact, hmmmm, actually it can be impossible! Unless you're a successful role model to them, and they somehow started to eat what you do. Rare miracle? But spinach has a very mild taste, so incorporating a large amount of leaves into this recipe doesn't affect the yummy taste of the fruit and dried fruits in it. Spinach is rich in vitamins A, C, and K, magnesium, iron, and manganese. Eating this leafy green veggie may benefit eye health, reduce oxidative stress, provide amino acids as building blocks for the proteins your body creates, and lots more...

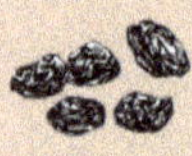

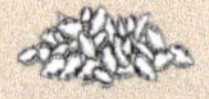

This is no ordinary cracker!

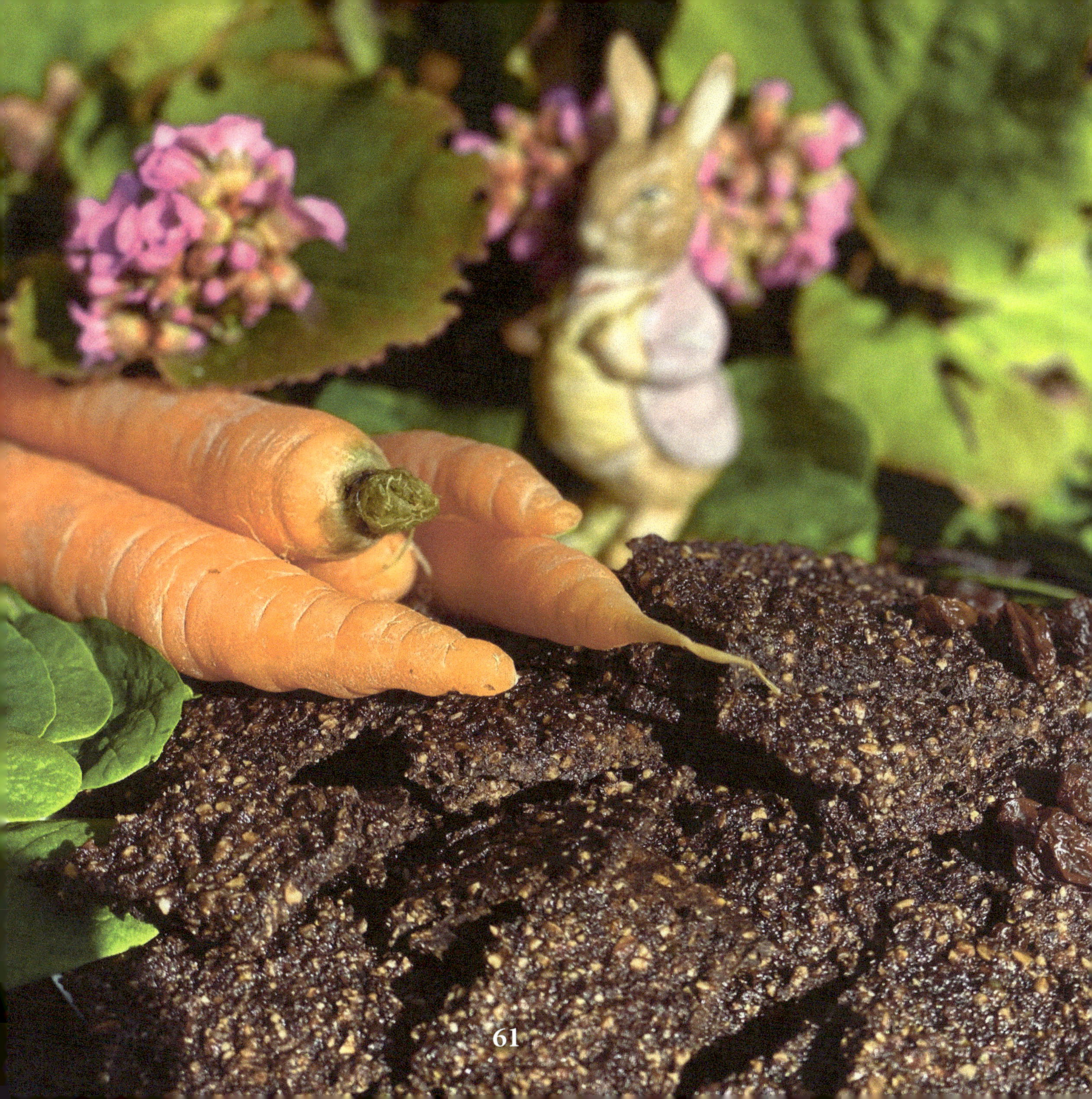

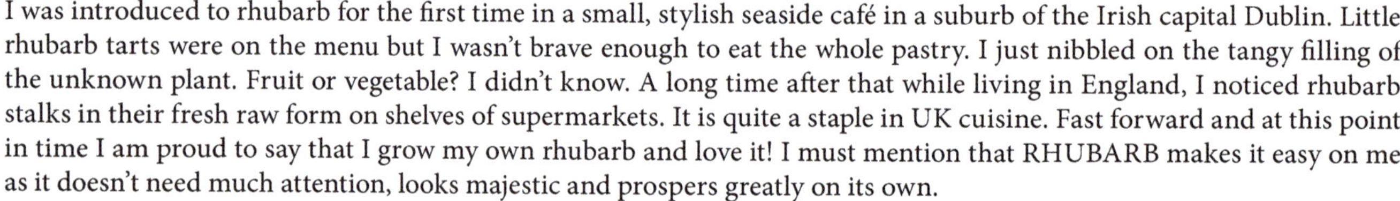

6

Ravishing RHUBARB

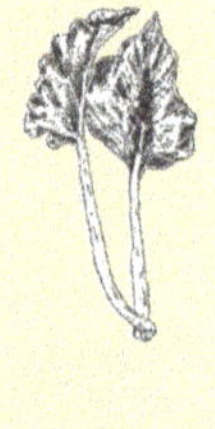

I was introduced to rhubarb for the first time in a small, stylish seaside café in a suburb of the Irish capital Dublin. Little rhubarb tarts were on the menu but I wasn't brave enough to eat the whole pastry. I just nibbled on the tangy filling of the unknown plant. Fruit or vegetable? I didn't know. A long time after that while living in England, I noticed rhubarb stalks in their fresh raw form on shelves of supermarkets. It is quite a staple in UK cuisine. Fast forward and at this point in time I am proud to say that I grow my own rhubarb and love it! I must mention that RHUBARB makes it easy on me as it doesn't need much attention, looks majestic and prospers greatly on its own.

Rhubarb is technically a vegetable but is legally considered a fruit (so says Mr. Google). In 1947, a New York court declared rhubarb a fruit... It is widely accepted that the stalks of rhubarb are edible as opposed to the big elephant-ear-shaped leaves. This is because the leaves (not the stalks in any significant amount) contain anthraquinone glycosides and oxalic acid. Oxalis acid consumed in higher doses promotes the formation of kidney stones.

The stalks are rich in vitamin C, vitamin B, and fiber. The roots of rhubarb were used in Chinese medicine for centuries, and believed to aid digestion.

This simple cracker recipe based on ravishing rhubarb turned out to be a big success in our 'village'. To make these crackers we need:

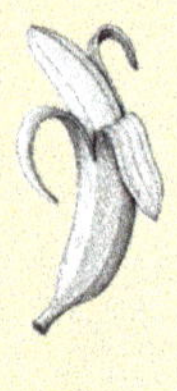

Ingredients

7 big rhubarb stalks (medium to big)

5 ripe bananas

250 g of raw pumpkin seeds

1 level tablespoon of raw coconut oil

Optional:
Strawberries
2 Parsnips
Apples/pineapple

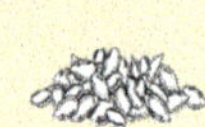

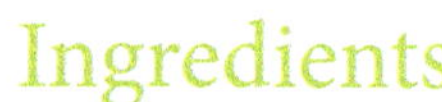

Process

Cut the rhubarb into smaller pieces and throw it in a blender. Add coconut oil and a cup of warm water as well as the parsnip/apples if you decide to include some in today's crackers. Run the blender a little until the veg and fruit are cut into smaller bits. Now you can add the bananas and pumpkin seeds, and blend until you like the smoothness of the raw cracker mass.

Spread the blended cracker mix evenly on the Teflex sheet placed on the dehydrator tray. Once spread evenly (think thin pizza crust) try to score the mix with the side of the spatula or blunt knife into slices or squares. If the consistency is still too runny – dehydrate it for a couple more hours and score it once the cracker mix thickens (meaning it's drier). Dry at 113 degrees F (45 degrees C) for approx. 5 hours. Check your crackers, flip them and peel off the sheets if possible. Peeling the crackers off sheets and leaving them on a bare mesh of dehydrator tray makes drying much faster – hence I try to peel the cracker mix from the sheets as soon as it's possible. Dehydrate for 4-5 hours more. Recheck the crackers and, if crispy-dry, store them in airtight boxes after a brief cooling down. If drying for a little longer is needed, you know what to do.

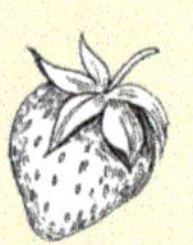

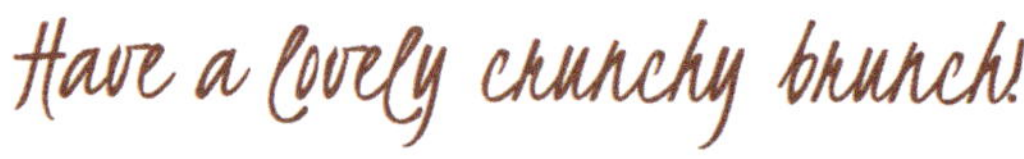

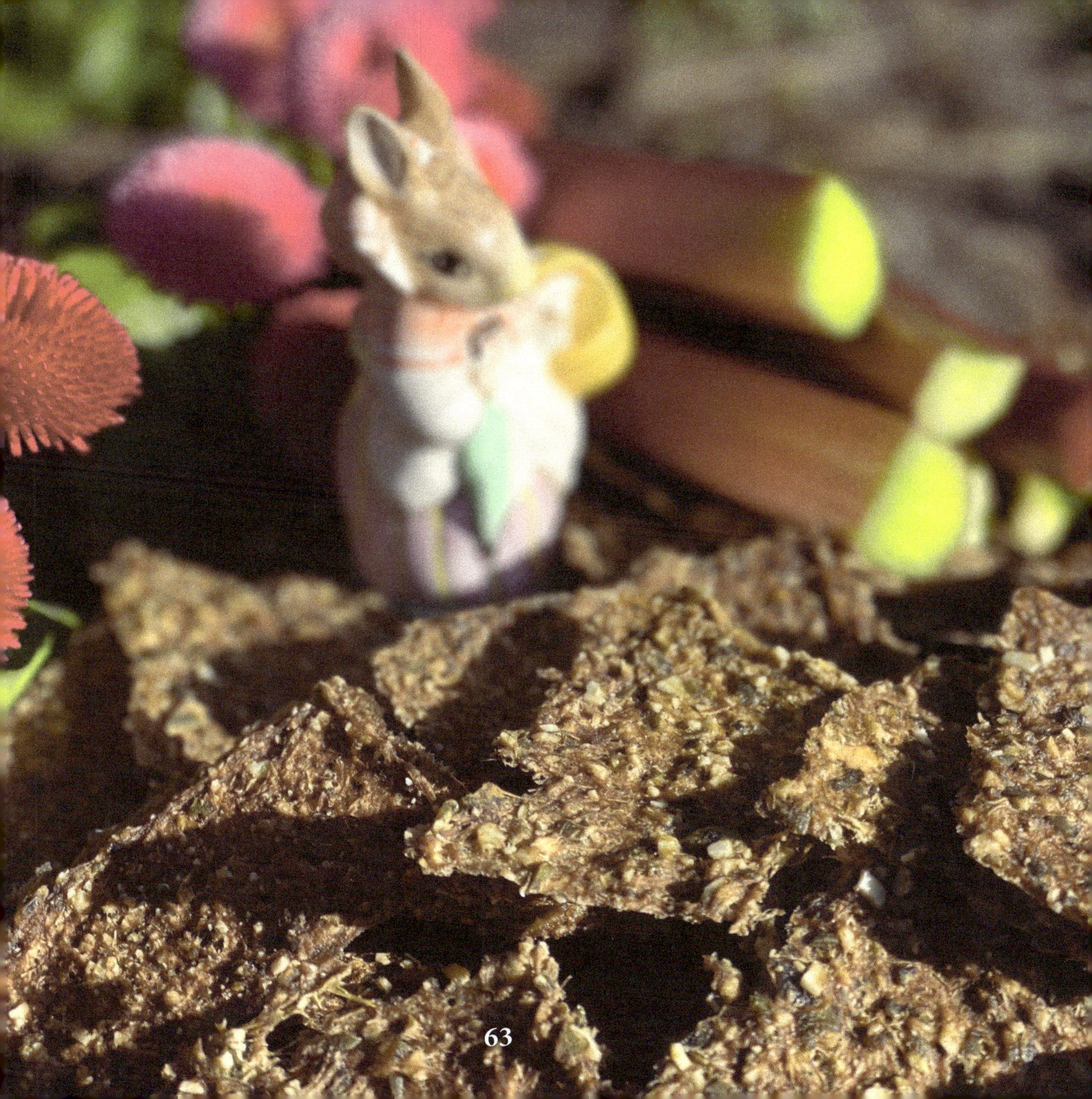

7

Very CHERRY

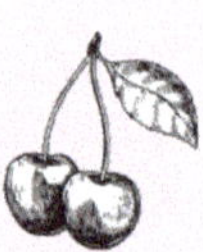

I did climb many trees as a kid… and as an adult too… some of the most memorable would be cherry trees. Sitting on a big comfy branch, observing the world from above, popping the juicy, crunchy fruit in my mouth, and yes – spitting out the pips. Maybe aiming to spit as far as possible or hit the target. Did you know it is actually an amateur sport? There are multiple international competitions for cherry pip spitting in countries such as the US, Canada, Germany, and France. (The world record by the way is almost 30 meters!)

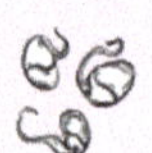

Anyway, who doesn't like fresh ripe cherries? Do you have a surplus harvest? Let's make crackers. This recipe takes a little bit of work, since the pips need to be removed from every single cherry. But that's an excuse for a fun family activity, the work necessary will be done in no time, and the health benefits are abundant.

Ingredients:

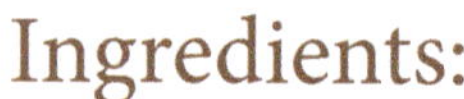

Approx. 1 kg of cherries (fresh or frozen*, make sure all the pips are out, we don't want to break a tooth) The amount of cherries can be even doubled for that extra cherry "cherriness"…

1 cup sprouted buckwheat (for more details about sprouting check page 20)

2 carrots

1 parsnip

1-2 ripe bananas

1 level tablespoon of raw coconut oil

Cup of raw seeds of your choice.

Optional:

*Add a little piece of **fresh beetroot** for vivid color.*
__Vanilla essence or pods__ for extra luxurious sweetness.
__Cocoa nibs or powder__ if you like life chocolatey.
__Lemon__ for a little tanginess.
__Orange__

Process

Place the carrots, parsnip, buckwheat sprouts and coconut oil into the blender with a cup of warm filtered water. Blend a little. Add seeds, bananas, and cherries and blend again until you like the texture.

Spread the blended cracker mix evenly on the Teflex sheet placed on the dehydrator tray. Once spread evenly (think thin pizza crust) try to score the mix with the side of the spatula or blunt knife into slices or squares. If the consistency is still too runny – dehydrate it for a couple more hours and score it once the cracker mix thickens (meaning it's drier). Dry at 113 degrees F (45 degrees C) for approx. 5 hours. Check your crackers, flip them and peel off the sheets if possible. Peeling the crackers off sheets and leaving them on a bare mesh of dehydrator tray makes drying much faster – hence I try to peel the cracker mix from the sheets as soon as it's possible. Dehydrate for 4-5 hours more. Recheck the crackers and, if crispy-dry, store them in airtight boxes after a brief cooling down. If drying for a little longer is needed, you know what to do.

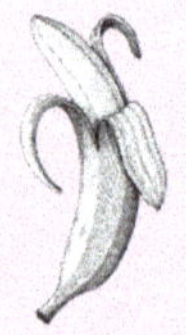
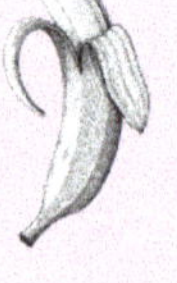
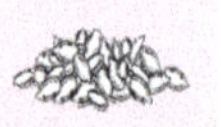

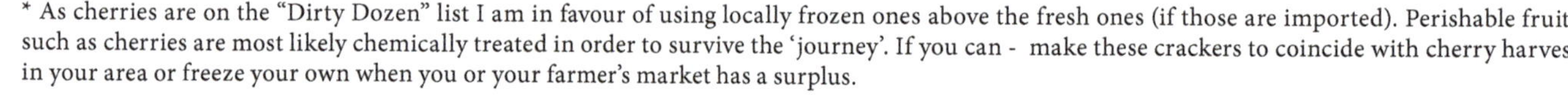

* As cherries are on the "Dirty Dozen" list I am in favour of using locally frozen ones above the fresh ones (if those are imported). Perishable fruits such as cherries are most likely chemically treated in order to survive the 'journey'. If you can - make these crackers to coincide with cherry harvest in your area or freeze your own when you or your farmer's market has a surplus.

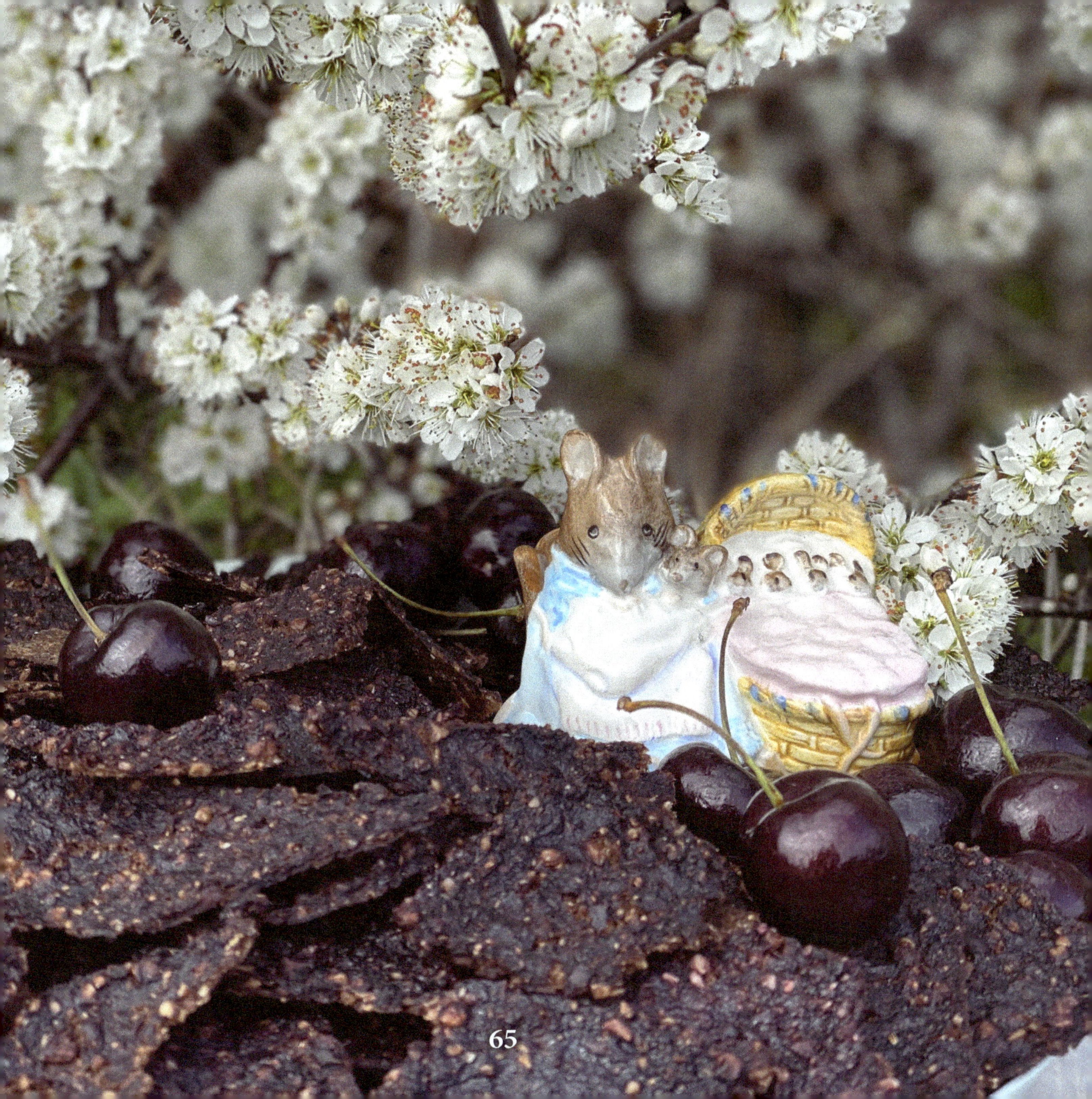

8

Luscious PEACH

My memories of peaches from childhood are divine. A couple of dozen peach trees in fields belonging to my sweetest grandma Maria bore fruit each summer. Peaches of all different types. Fragrant and juicy. They could reach the size of a big orange when the weather was kind. My little sister and I would sit on a bench under a huge old walnut tree with the sweet juice dripping from our hands, elbows, cheeks, and our noses all sticky. Those peaches were just irresistible. I am sure we often lost count of how many each one of us had eaten in a day.

For this recipe use only very ripe peaches, approx. 2 kg. Halve them and remove the stones. I also include:

Ingredients:

2 kg peaches

2 ripe bananas

2 apples

A couple of parsnips

½ peeled lemon, seeds removed

1 level tablespoon of raw virgin coconut oil

300 g of mixed raw seeds

Optional:

*Swap parsnips for **carrots or carrot pulp** left over from juicing*

Process

Place the parsnips, lemon, apples, coconut oil, and up to one cup of lukewarm filtered water in the blender. Blend until the parsnip is homogenized. Add the peaches, bananas, and seeds and blend again. Use the tamper in your blender to help the mass blend equally, adjusting the speed downward if needed. Blend until you like the structure of the cracker mass.

Spread the blended cracker mix evenly on the Teflex sheet placed on the dehydrator tray. Once spread evenly (think thin pizza crust) try to score the mix with the side of the spatula or blunt knife into slices or squares. If the consistency is still too runny – dehydrate it for a couple more hours and score it once the cracker mix thickens (meaning it's drier). Dry at 113 degrees F (45 degrees C) for approx. 5 hours. Check your crackers, flip them and peel off the sheets if possible. Peeling the crackers off sheets and leaving them on a bare mesh of dehydrator tray makes drying much faster – hence I try to peel the cracker mix from the sheets as soon as it's possible. Dehydrate for 4-5 hours more. Recheck the crackers and, if crispy-dry, store them in airtight boxes after a brief cooling down. If drying for a little longer is needed, you know what to do.

Oh my sweet crackers!

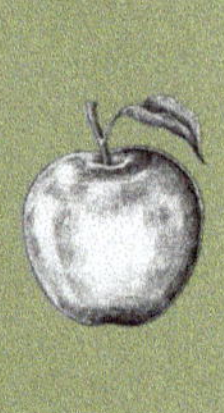
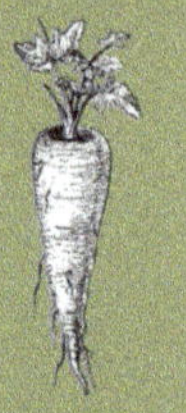
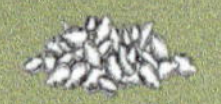

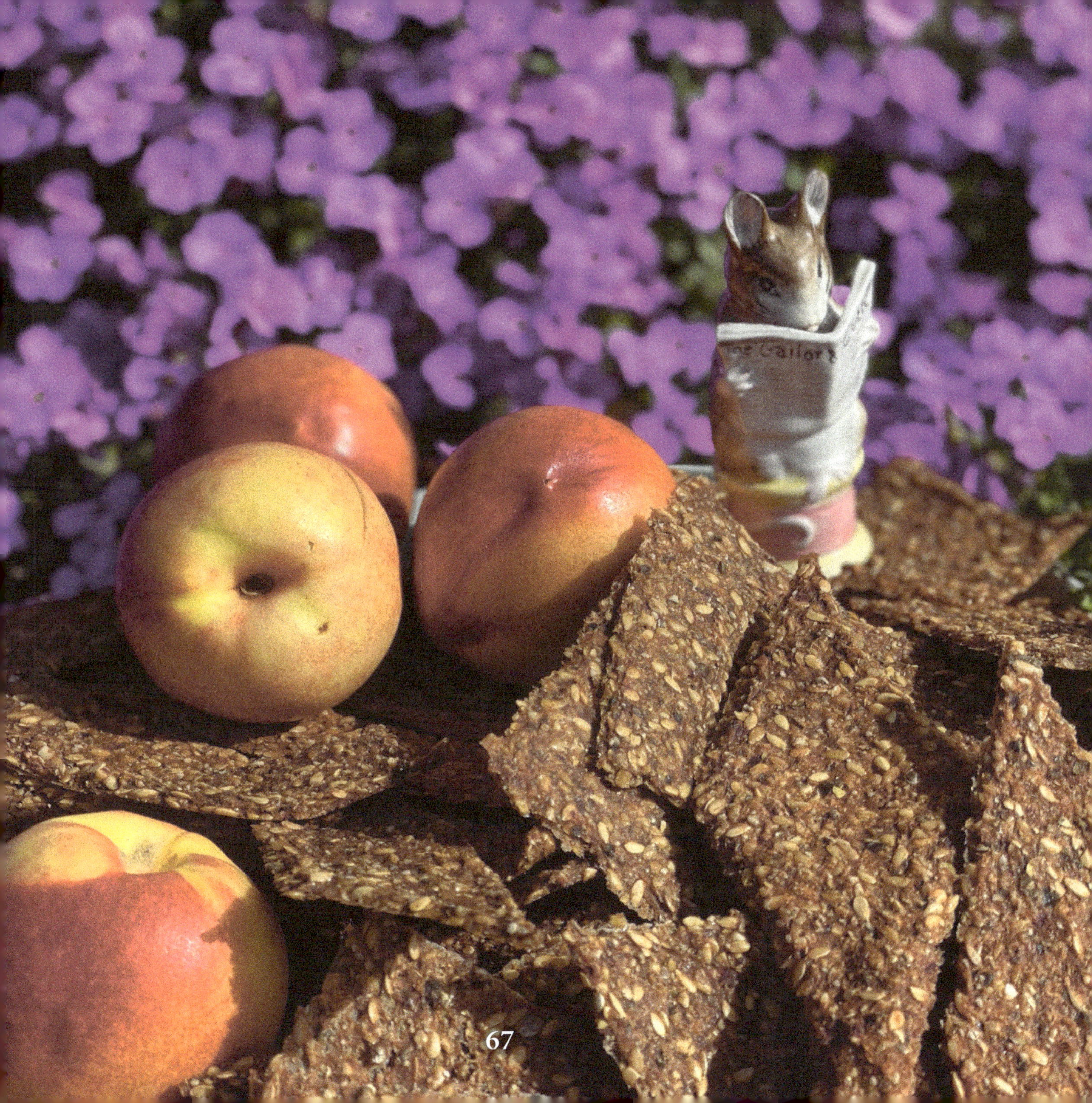

9

Knockout KIWI

Kiwi fruit is native to central and eastern China. Traditionally in China, kiwi fruit was not eaten for pleasure but was given as medicine to children to help them grow and to women who had given birth to help them recover. Luckily nowadays this wonderful (rich in vitamin C & K) fruit is available all around the world.

Hopefully, you and your kids often enjoy some ripe juicy kiwis. By the way, did you know the whole fruit, including the skin, is suitable for human consumption? Just wash the fruit very well and make sure they are free of chemicals. Also, wait until your kiwi fruit is really truly ripe. (To help them ripen — place in a bag with a banana, apple, or pear.)

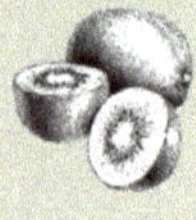

Ingredients:

As many very ripe kiwis as you can spare: let's say 1-2 kilograms

2 parsnips

2 ripe bananas

Juice from 1/2 lemon

Vanilla pod

Raw seeds of your choice- I like to use a mix of chia seeds and sunflower seeds, sometimes yellow flax seeds (250 g)

1 level tablespoon of raw coconut oil

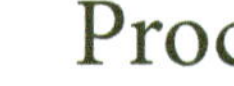

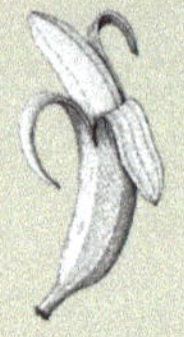

Process

Place all ingredients in a blender together with upto one cup of warm filtered water. If needed, add little bit of warm filtered water for easier blending. If your kiwis are truly ripe and soft, you may not need to add water at all. Blend until you like the texture.

Spread the blended cracker mix evenly on the Teflex sheet placed on the dehydrator tray. Once spread evenly (think thin pizza crust) try to score the mix with the side of the spatula or blunt knife into slices or squares. If the consistency is still too runny – dehydrate it for a couple more hours and score it once the cracker mix thickens (meaning it's drier). Dry at 113 degrees F (45 degrees C) for approx. 5 hours. Check your crackers, flip them and peel off the sheets if possible. Peeling the crackers off sheets and leaving them on a bare mesh of dehydrator tray makes drying much faster – hence I try to peel the cracker mix from the sheets as soon as it's possible. Dehydrate for 4-5 hours more. Recheck the crackers and, if crispy-dry, store them in airtight boxes after a brief cooling down. If drying for a little longer is needed, you know what to do.

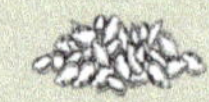

Cracker snacks are back!

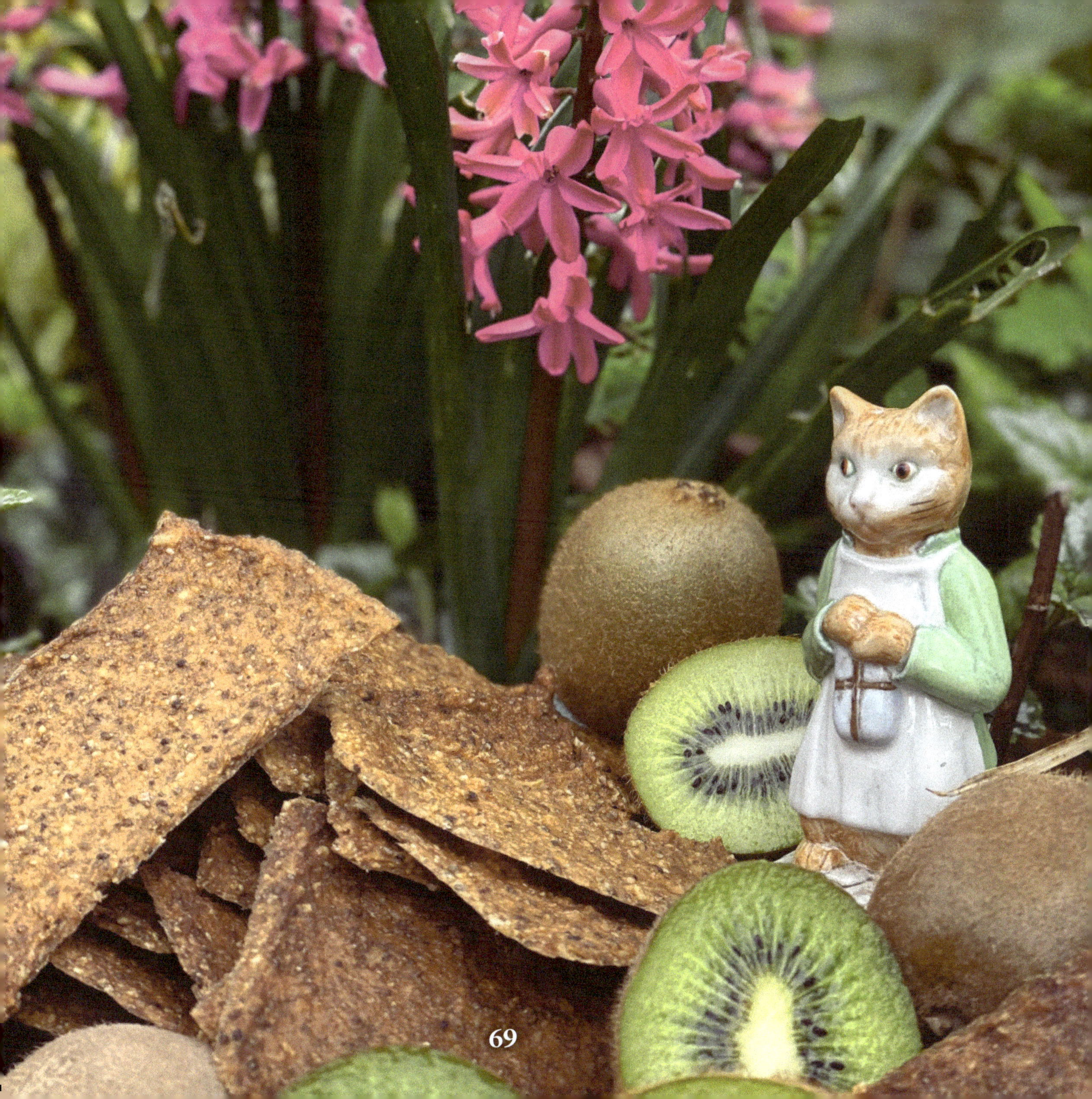

10

Brainy PRUNES and WALNUTS

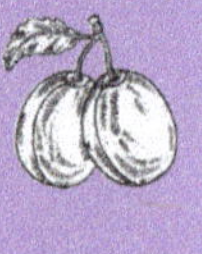
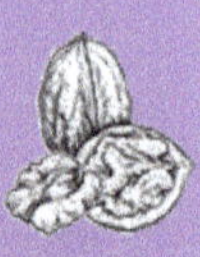

Another combo I love. Walnuts are one of the healthiest nuts. Great for the brain, heart, and immunity health and development – as they are a good source of plant-based omega-3 fatty acids, folate, vitamin B1 and B6. Walnuts are also packed with essential minerals like magnesium, potassium, calcium, zinc, selenium, etc., which are required for the optimal growth of your child. Calcium strengthens the bones, while iron manages hemoglobin levels. The potassium and sodium in walnuts help balance electrolytes, and phosphorous aids digestion, cell repair, and protein generation in your child's growing body.

Walnuts contain melatonin, which helps induce sleep and regulates body functions during sleep. Sleep is necessary for children since most of the growth happens when they enter deep sleep.

Walnuts also contain high-quality vegetable protein, fiber, and compounds like tocopherols, phytosterols, phenolic compounds, and other vitamins such as vitamin A, C, E, and K, which directly benefit the child's growth.

Prunes and plums? Feel free to use either. Both will work very well as long they are ripened.

They are rich in fiber and contain sorbitol – which both help relieve constipation. Prunes may promote bone health, containing minerals such as potassium, copper, manganese, vitamins A, C, K, antioxidants (polyphenols, anthocyanins).

Enough of the theory, let's get crackering.

Ingredients:

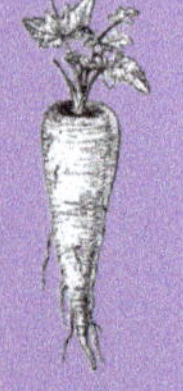

1-2 kg of ripe prunes/plums

500 g raw walnuts (best soak them for a couple of hours before using)

3 parsnips

2 ripe bananas

2 apples

1 level tablespoon of raw coconut oil

Optional:

Cinnamon

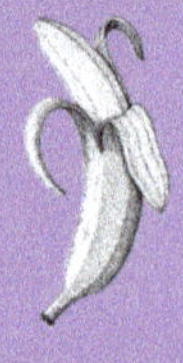

Process

Place all the ingredients into the blender. I like to blend the parsnips, apples, bananas, coconut oil and a splash of water first. Blend for a minute or two. Only then add the walnuts and prunes, and blend again. This way little bits of nuts and prunes/plums remain visible in the final texture of the cracker.

Spread the blended cracker mix evenly on the Teflex sheet placed on the dehydrator tray. Once spread evenly (think thin pizza crust) try to score the mix with the side of the spatula or blunt knife into slices or squares. If the consistency is still too runny – dehydrate it for a couple more hours and score it once the cracker mix thickens (meaning it's drier). Dry at 113 degrees F (45 degrees C) for approx. 5 hours. Check your crackers, flip them and peel off the sheets if possible. Peeling the crackers off sheets and leaving them on a bare mesh of dehydrator tray makes drying much faster – hence I try to peel the cracker mix from the sheets as soon as it's possible. Dehydrate for 4-5 hours more. Recheck the crackers and, if crispy-dry, store them in airtight boxes after a brief cooling down. If drying for a little longer is needed, you know what to do.

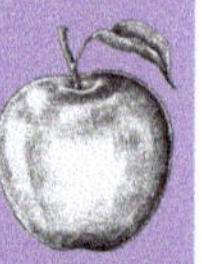

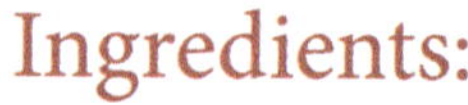

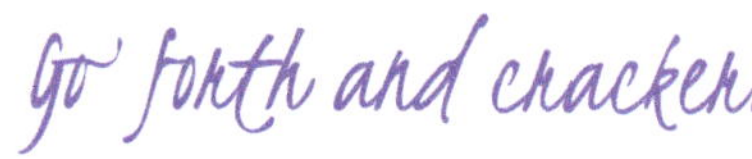

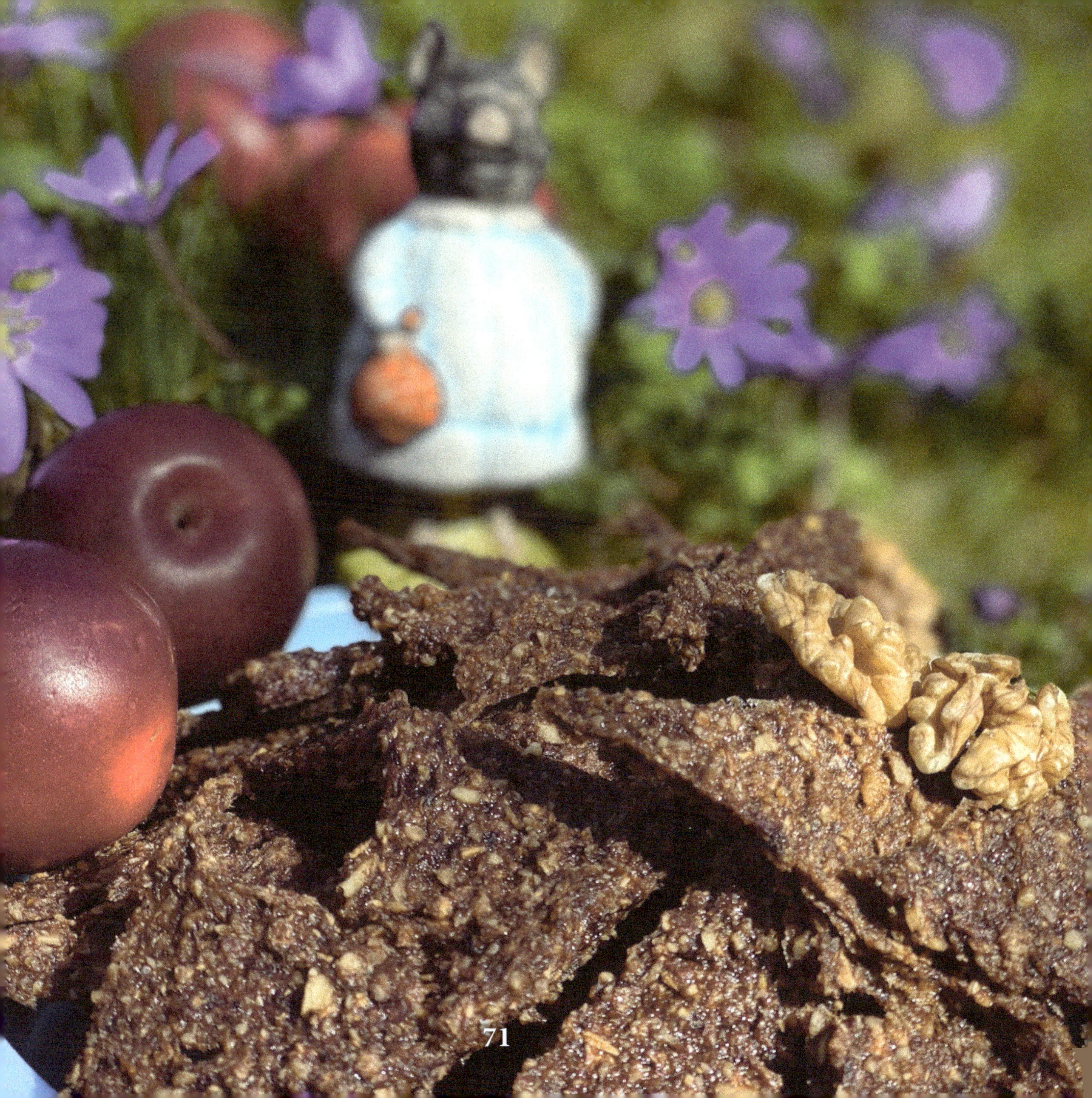

11

Magnificent MANGO

I was lucky to spend some amazing months in the smallest (by area) state of India – Goa. Magical memories. Beaches, fruit, beautiful people...

Goa's rich culture has a unique connection to delicious mango varieties like nowhere else. The mango season in Goa lasts from February/March to the end of the summer.

Goa is home to a couple of hundred varieties of mangos. So many different tastes, textures, sizes, and names that most of us haven't even heard of (let alone tasted). To witness the buzz of fruit markets in this season is an unforgettable experience, especially for mango lovers.

If you are from any beautiful part of this world where the climate is favorable to growing mangos, or if perhaps your local fruit shop has some in stock, please try this cracker recipe.

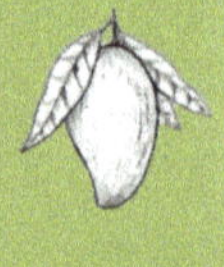

Ingredients:

5-7 big ripe mangos (more than 7 is fine too)

1-2 parsnips

3-5 carrots

1/3 small pumpkin (or butternut squash)

300 g mixed raw seeds (sunflower, sesame, hemp, flax)

1 level tablespoon of raw coconut oil

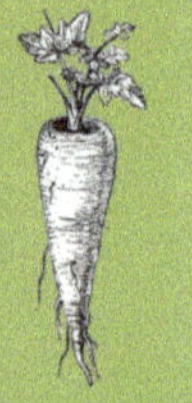

Optional:

Ripe banana

Lemon/lime juice *for an extra tangy kick*

Dried unsweetened mango *(300g)*

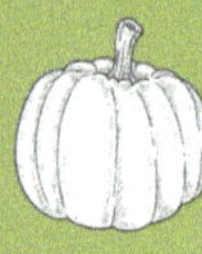

Process

Clean and peel the mangos, remove the stones and place them in the blender. Add into the blender the carrots, parsnips and pumpkin – all peeled and cut into 2-3 cm pieces. Add the coconut oil and whizz the blender for a minute or two. If the mangos are truly ripe, you shouldn't need to add water to this recipe. (If you sense your blender is 'struggling' then feel free to add some water for easier blending.) Now add the seeds and all the optional ingredients you chose to use (if any) and blend again until you like the texture of the cracker mix.

Spread the blended cracker mix evenly on the Teflex sheet placed on the dehydrator tray. Once spread evenly (think thin pizza crust) try to score the mix with the side of the spatula or blunt knife into slices or squares. If the consistency is still too runny – dehydrate it for a couple more hours and score it once the cracker mix thickens (meaning it's drier). Dry at 113 degrees F (45 degrees C) for approx. 5 hours. Check your crackers, flip them and peel off the sheets if possible. Peeling the crackers off sheets and leaving them on a bare mesh of dehydrator tray makes drying much faster – hence I try to peel the cracker mix from the sheets as soon as it's possible. Dehydrate for 4-5 hours more. Recheck the crackers and, if crispy-dry, store them in airtight boxes after a brief cooling down. If drying for a little longer is needed, you know what to do.

Mango is an amazing fruit, rich in vitamins vitamin C, A, E, B6, B9...

It also contains vitamins K, B3, B5, B2, B1, fiber and minerals, especially copper, along with potassium, manganese, magnesium...

As with every fruit I mentioned so far, it is important to find and use only ripe and organic ones! These crackers may not turn out magnificent at all if the mango is not ripe...

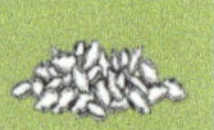

Time for not doing – just crunching!

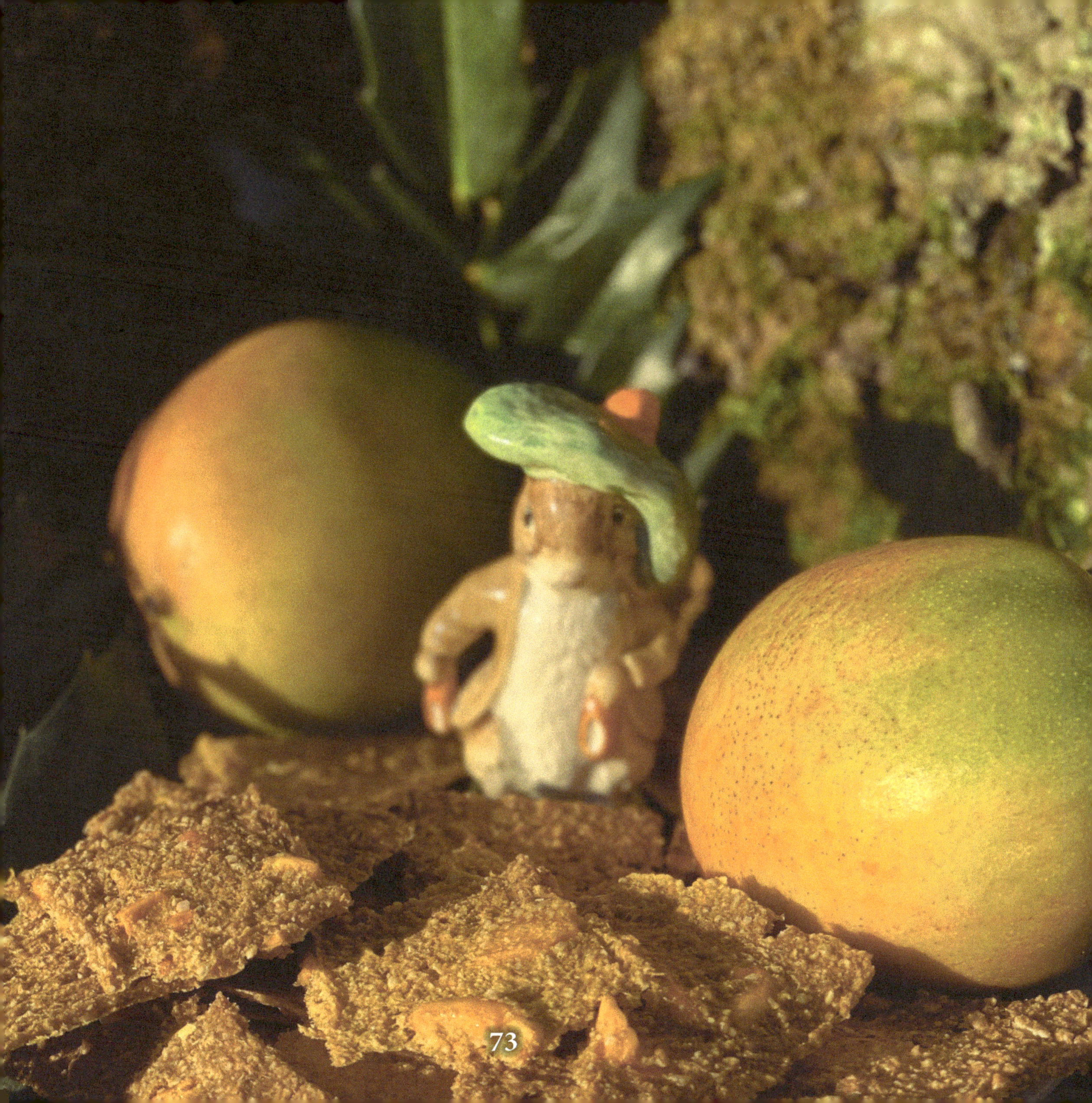

12

Tempting ORANGE

When I see a beautiful golden orange I think of the warm sun.

Walking in orange plantations, admiring the flowering trees, taking deep breaths of air filled with fragrant orange blossom scent makes me appreciate the magic of life.

The color of this luscious fruit makes me HAPPY...

Here is the simple recipe:

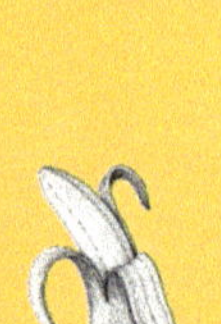

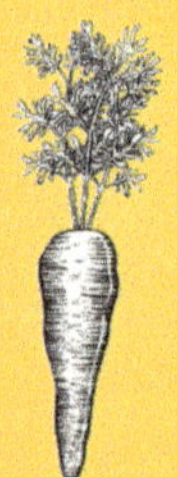

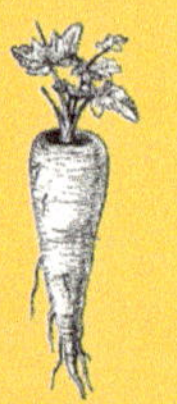

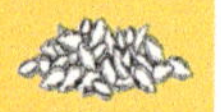

Ingredients:

6-8 big oranges (use tangerines if you prefer)

2-3 ripe bananas

A couple of whole carrots or leftovers from carrot juicing

2-3 parsnips

1 level tablespoon of raw coconut oil

Your preferred combo of mixed raw seeds 300-400 g

Process

Peel the oranges and remove the pips. Place them in the blender together with the parsnips, carrots, coconut oil. Blend until the carrots and parsnips are chopped into small pieces. Then add seeds and bananas and blend more until the cracker mass has a texture you like.

Spread the blended cracker mix evenly on the Teflex sheet placed on the dehydrator tray. Once spread evenly (think thin pizza crust) try to score the mix with the side of the spatula or blunt knife into slices or squares. If the consistency is still too runny – dehydrate it for a couple more hours and score it once the cracker mix thickens (meaning it's drier). Dry at 113 degrees F (45 degrees C) for approx. 5 hours. Check your crackers, flip them and peel off the sheets if possible. Peeling the crackers off sheets and leaving them on a bare mesh of dehydrator tray makes drying much faster – hence I try to peel the cracker mix from the sheets as soon as it's possible. Dehydrate for 4-5 hours more. Recheck the crackers and, if crispy-dry, store them in airtight boxes after a brief cooling down. If drying for a little longer is needed, you know what to do.

Orange crackers will have a mild pleasant taste.

It is not only the vitamin C that we all know about that oranges contain. Healthy carotenoids, flavonoids, pectins, fiber are some goodies to mention, great to include in yours and your family's diet.

If you desire a little bit of fire: Try adding some chili powder and possibly cocoa to the mixture. The crackers will be a nice chili-orange-chocolate.

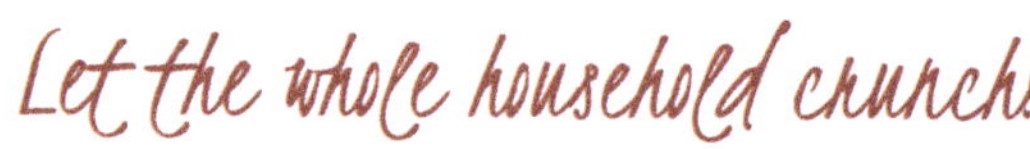

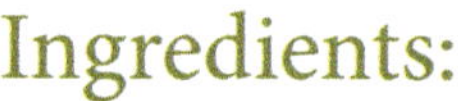

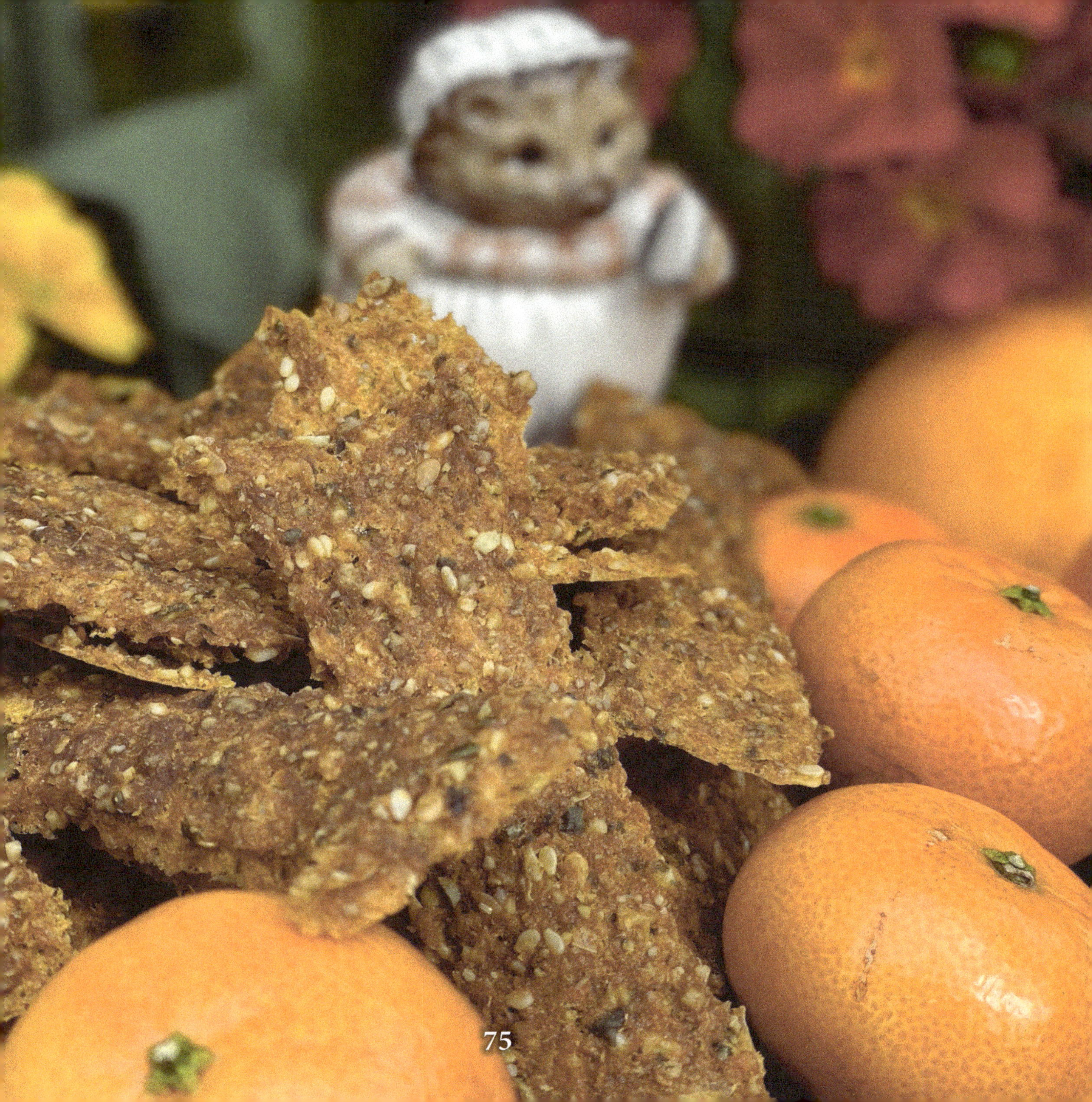

13

Bright PEAR with golden RAISINS and FLAXSEEDS

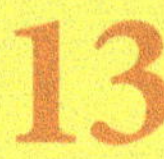

This seems to be many kids' favorite — maybe because of the mild taste, or soft chewy texture, reminding them of comfort snacking on raisins.

Can you lay your hands on organic local pears? Juicy or a bit crunchy, all are fine. The important thing for this recipe is for them to be ripe.

I like the proverb: "WHEN THE PEAR IS RIPE IT FALLS BY ITSELF".

It reminds me to practice the virtue of patience in every aspect of life.

Thank you for your patience in getting to the list of ingredients:

Ingredients:

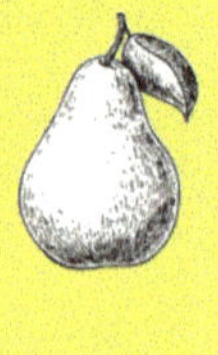

4-7 Pear-fectly imperfect ripe organic PEARS

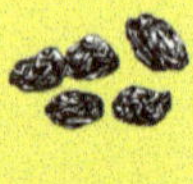

Bag of golden raisins (approx. 500 g)

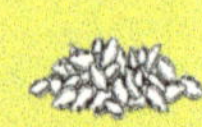

300-400 g of golden flaxseeds

2-3 parsnips

1-2 ripe bananas

Juice from ½ lemon (can be more if you prefer a nice tangy final taste)

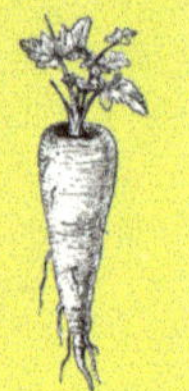

1 level tablespoon of raw coconut oil

Optional:

Vanilla pod or essence

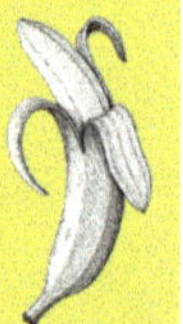

Process

Remove the cores from all the pears, and place them in the blender together with the parsnips, lemon juice, coconut oil, and a cup of warm water.

Blend until the parsnips are chopped into small bits.

Add the bananas, yellow flaxseeds, and golden raisins and blend again until you achieve the texture you like. Maybe experiment if it is your first time making this recipe to get the texture your kids will truly like and enjoy the most. What I mean is to stop blending when you can still see some bits of raisins in the cracker mix and remove just enough of the mix from the blender to spread on one silicone sheet.

After that continue blending – your cracker mix will become less 'grainy' – spread it on the second silicone sheet. After that try to blend the remaining cracker mix a little further. Maybe until totally smooth...

Try to score the cracker mix with the side of the spatula or blunt knife into slices or squares. If the consistency is still too runny – dehydrate it for a couple more hours and score it once it's thickened (meaning it's drier). Dry at 113 degrees F (45 degrees C) for approx. 5 hours. Check your crackers, flip them and peel off the sheets if possible. Peeling the crackers off sheets and leaving them on a bare mesh of dehydrator tray makes drying much faster – hence I try to peel the blended cracker mix from the sheets as soon as it's possible. Dehydrate for 4-5 hours more. Recheck the crackers and, if crispy-dry, store them in airtight boxes after a brief cooling down. If drying for a little longer is needed, you know what to do.

Tip: For a nice variation of this recipe — add cinnamon

Enjoy!

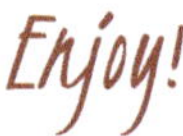

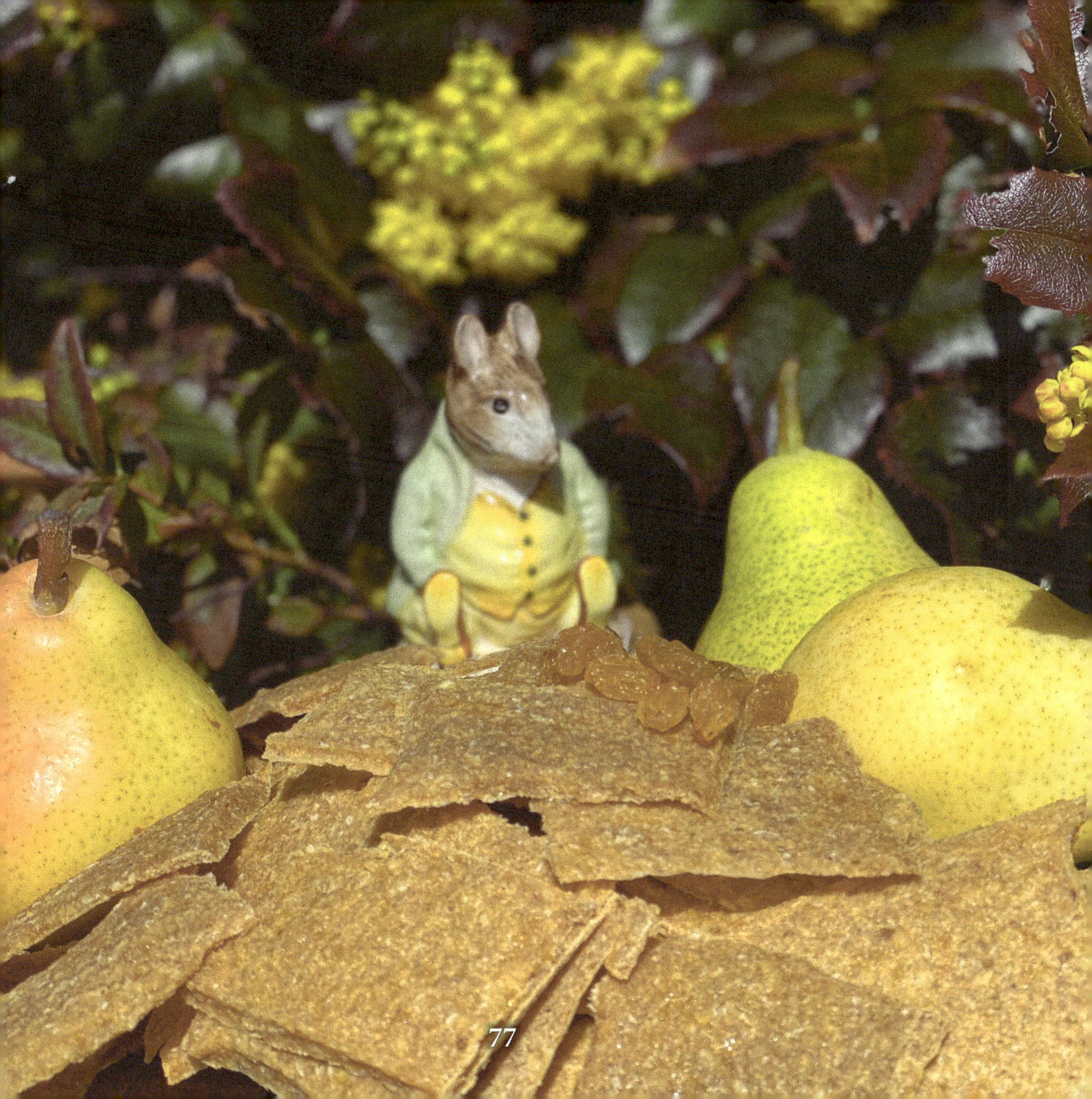

14

Fabulous FIGS and POPPY SEEDS

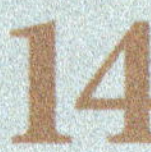

My sister loves pie with poppy seeds and apple filling. It is more a puff pastry strudel than a pie. A traditional baked delicacy in the place where we come from. I would share a picture here but that would be way off track from my clean and healthy snacking mission!

I got inspired by the thought of her beloved treat, added my favorite dried fruit to the combo, and voilà — this fabulous figs and poppy seeds recipe was born.

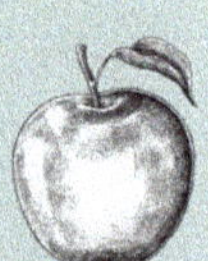

Ingredients:

Pulp leftovers from apple and carrots juicing

Or

3-4 apples and 2 carrots

2 parsnips

1 -2 ripe bananas

1 level tablespoon of raw coconut oil

1-2 kg of ripe fresh figs (substitute with approx. 500 g of dried figs)

300 g of dried 'washed' poppy seeds

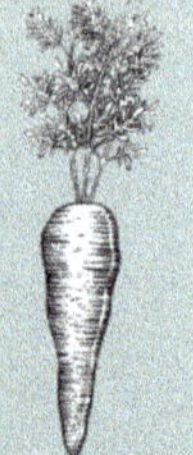

Commercially-sold poppy seeds are usually 'washed,' hence safe to eat for kids. Make sure you source poppy seeds from a safe shop.

Optional:

Chia seeds

Process

Place all the ingredients into the blender with up to a cup of warm filtered water. Blend until the texture seems right and is even overall.

Spread the blended cracker mix evenly on the Teflex sheet placed on the dehydrator tray. Once spread evenly (think thin pizza crust) try to score the mix with the side of the spatula or blunt knife into slices or squares. If the consistency is still too runny – dehydrate it for a couple more hours and score it once the cracker mix thickens (meaning it's drier). Dry at 113 degrees F (45 degrees C) for approx. 5 hours. Check your crackers, flip them and peel off the sheets if possible. Peeling the crackers off sheets and leaving them on a bare mesh of dehydrator tray makes drying much faster – hence I try to peel the cracker mix from the sheets as soon as it's possible. Dehydrate for 4-5 hours more. Recheck the crackers and, if crispy-dry, store them in airtight boxes after a brief cooling down. If drying for a little longer is needed, you know what to do.

Poppy seeds are a great source of calcium and iron. (By the way I recommend adding milk made from poppy seeds to the diet of people who suffer from osteoporosis.) For growing kids, calcium, iron, and other minerals (such as copper manganese), as well omega 6 and omega 9 fatty acids, fiber, and antioxidants contained in poppy seeds are needed for healthy growth and development.

Figs, quite apart from being super yummy, are a great healthy fruit, aiding digestion, insulin control, immunity, and general health…

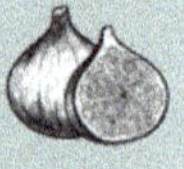

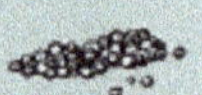

Ready steady cracker!

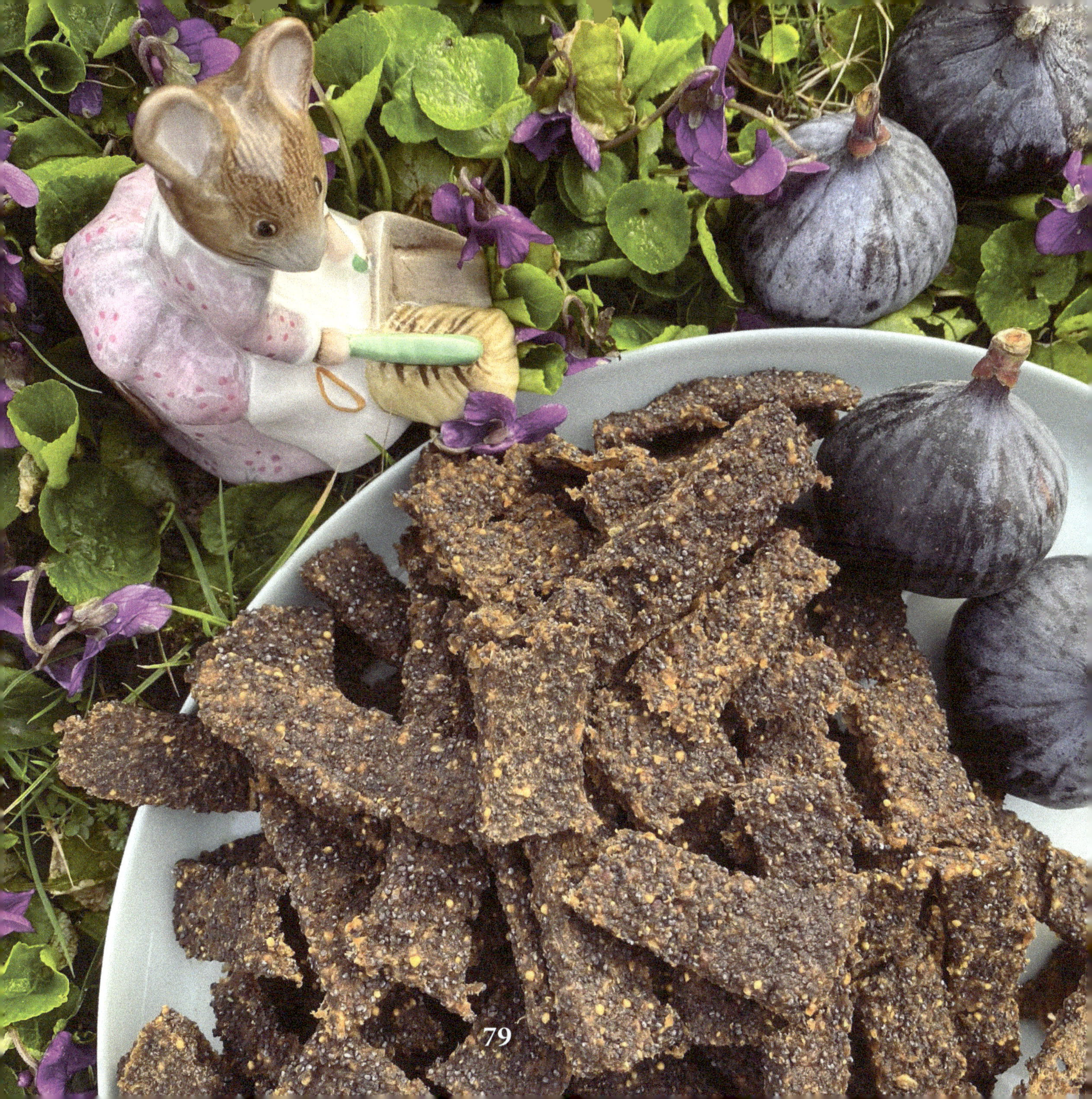

15

Happy STRAWBERRY

We love strawberries...

However, strawberries make it year after year to the top of the "dirty dozen" list.

In 2021, strawberries actually continued to lead the list of fruits and veggies that contain the highest levels of pesticides, followed by spinach, a trio of greens – kale, collard, and mustard – nectarines, apples, and grapes, according to the Environmental Working Group.*

Even though I love to remain positive — starting this page with the warning is intentional. I want every parent to understand the importance of sourcing only clean and safe produce. If you can, try to start growing your own food. It can become a very rewarding endeavor, I promise you. Strawberries in particular are easy to grow and can bear fruit twice a year. And yes, you will not have to worry about chemicals in and on them. (If your soil and the water you use are clean.)

Try to plant new plants from existing plant runners or if you have the patience, grow them from seed. By the way, the average strawberry has approx. 200 seeds on it. That's potentially lots of new baby plants.

This low in calories, high in vitamin C, manganese, and potassium fruit plant will bear fruit soon enough.

For this fragrant, happy recipe loved by many we need:

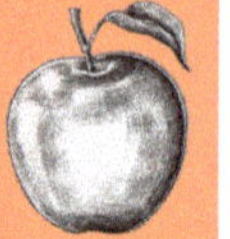
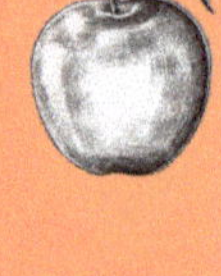
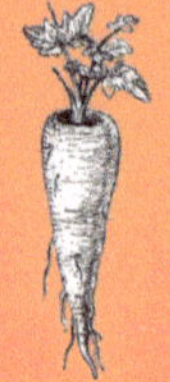
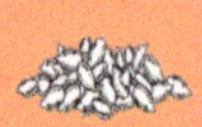

Ingredients:

1-2 kg of strawberries (more is better here, let's just say fill at least ½ of a blender with ripe and organic strawberries)

1-2 apples

1-2 parsnips

Chia seeds & sunflower seeds & hemp seed (all raw with the total weight of the seed mix approx 300g)

1 level tablespoon of raw coconut oil

Optional:

Carrots, ripe bananas, lemon juice

Process

Tip for very naughty parents — add a 'squirt' of strawberry cordial to enhance the strawberry flavor. This makes a difference especially if the strawberries you're using are from a big supermarket chain. They usually aren't as fragrant as the "real deal" I get in my own garden.

I like to blend all the ingredients first, apart from half the total amount of strawberries and seeds. Only after everything else is blended will I add the rest of the strawberries and seeds and whizz my blender a little more. This is to preserve the bigger bits of strawberries (and seeds) in the final cracker for me to admire. It is also absolutely fine to place all the ingredients in the blender at the beginning of the process if you wish.

Continue with the METHOD on pages 40-41

Tip for BRAVE parents — add a handful of very young strawberry leaves to part of your strawberry cracker mix for extra protein and healing power. The taste of young strawberry leaves is not too strong, and will not compete with the fragrant fruit flavor.

Let's have a berry happy day!

---

* Avoiding pesticides is especially critical for babies and children, because of the damage they can cause to the developing brain. Studies have found an increase in IQ loss and intellectual disability in children with exposure to organophosphates, a common class of pesticides.

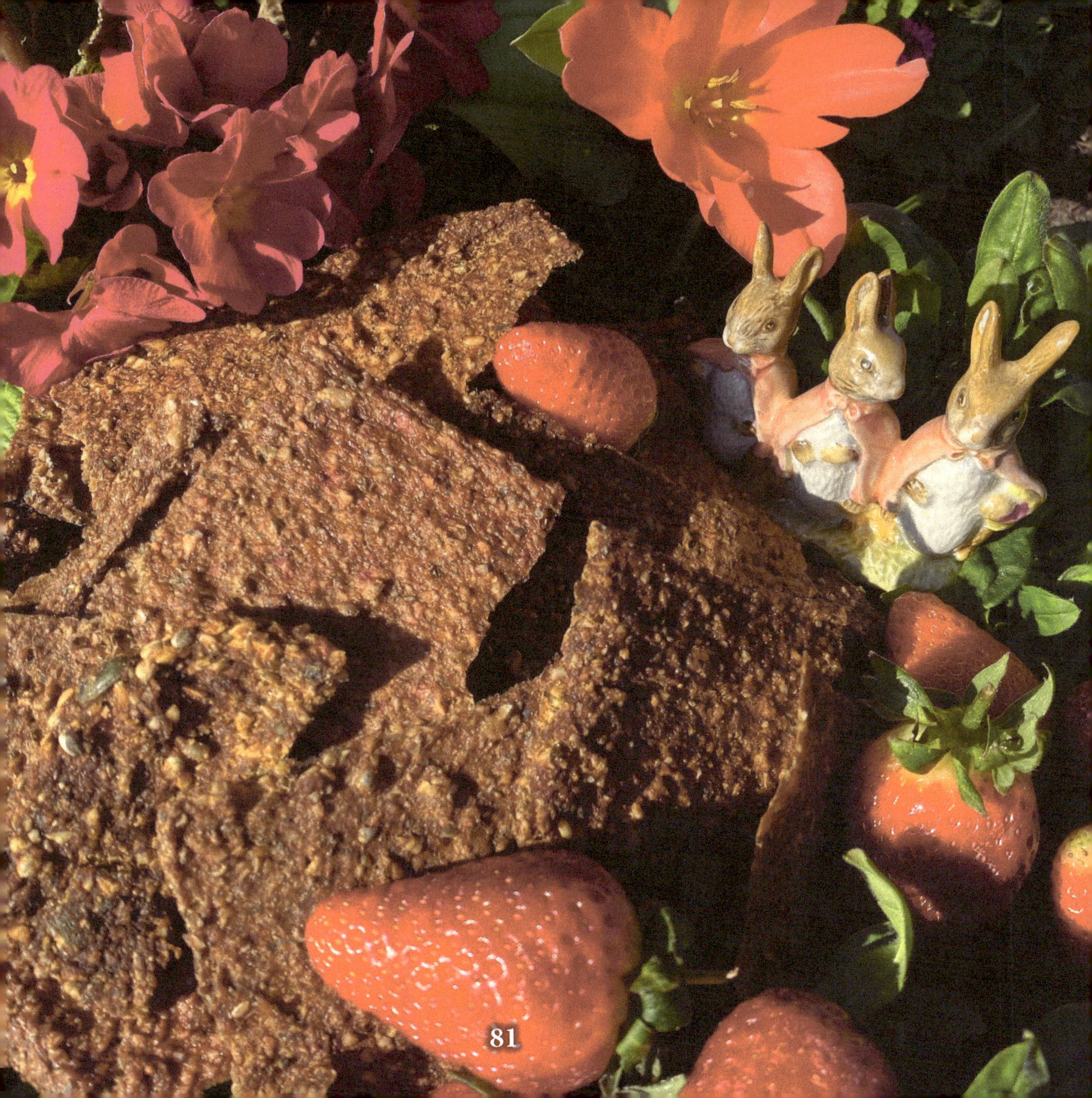

16

Delightful GINGERBREAD

The history of gingerbread goes back centuries. There are countless variations of this popular aromatic treat in countries around the world and these are often associated with Christmas.

What most of them have in common is the signature spice combo of ginger and cinnamon, often with added dried cloves and local honey.

Can you imagine gingerbread weighing 651 kg? (1,435 lbs) Giant, right? In Oslo, Norway in 2009 the world's largest gingerbread man was made, according to the Guinness Book of World Records.

Our version of a cracker with a flavor reminiscent of gingerbread will be light and easily fit into your kid's pocket. And of course, it will be clean, healthy, gluten-and-preservative-free, and safe to eat.

Ingredients:

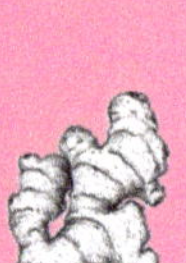

Ginger and cinnamon (add the amount you think your kids can handle. This will depend on their age and possibly their inner culinary adventurer. I would use one heaped tablespoon of cinnamon and a chunk of fresh ginger as big as table-tennis-ball.)

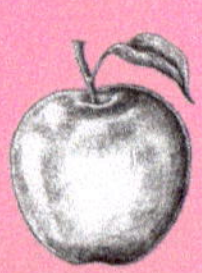

I usually use fresh ginger root, but dried is fine as well. Safely sourced whole cinnamon bark is a good bet, you can grind it at home, or just throw it as a whole piece of bark in a blender. A powerful blender will finish the job.)

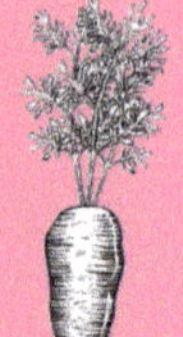

3-5 apples

2-4 carrots

3-5 parsnips

2 ripe bananas

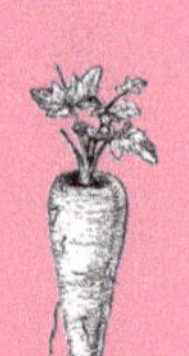

300 g raw mixed seeds or just single seeds (for example raw sunflower seeds)

1 level tablespoon of raw coconut oil

100g local farmer's honey

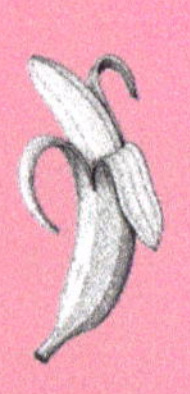

Optional:

Cloves, swap apples for **pears**

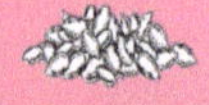

Process

Blend all the ingredients in your blender with a cup of filtered water (add more water if needed). Stop blending only once you are happy with the texture of the mixture.

Spread the blended cracker mix evenly on the Teflex sheet placed on the dehydrator tray. Once spread evenly (think thin pizza crust) try to score the mix with the spatula or blunt knife into shapes you like. You can also attempt to create shapes of gingerbread men if you feel artistic and/or have the right cookie cutter.

If the consistency is still too runny – dehydrate it for a couple more hours and score it once the cracker mix thickens (meaning it's drier). Dry at 113 degrees F (45 degrees C) for approx. 5 hours. Check your crackers, flip them and peel off the sheets if possible. Peeling the crackers off sheets and leaving them on a bare mesh of dehydrator tray makes drying much faster – hence I try to peel the cracker mix from the sheets as soon as it's possible. Dehydrate for 4-5 hours more. Recheck the crackers and, if crispy-dry, store them in airtight boxes after a brief cooling down. If drying for a little longer is needed, you know what to do.

If you need more reasons to try these (other than the tasty crispy festive HEALTHY treat in your cookie jar), here is the rundown of some of the potential medicinal effects spices in your crackers can offer:

Both, fresh and dried ginger roots have therapeutic properties for digestion, hypertension and headaches. For kids who are constipated or suffer from gas and bloated tummy, ginger can help to "move" things. Ginger is excellent for nausea and motion sickness so pack and take these crackers on your sea, road, and air trips too. Ginger promotes the secretion of digestive juices, improves appetite, alleviates pain, and has an overall impressive anti-inflammatory effect.

Cinnamon is much more than just a great-tasting pastry spice. It helps counter spikes in sugar levels when one eats sweets, has a strong fungicide, antibacterial, anti-parasitic effect, and helps stimulate blood circulation. It also helps to relieve cramps, colic, stress, anxiety and general body pains, diarrhea, and gas...

Ho-ho-ho crackers!

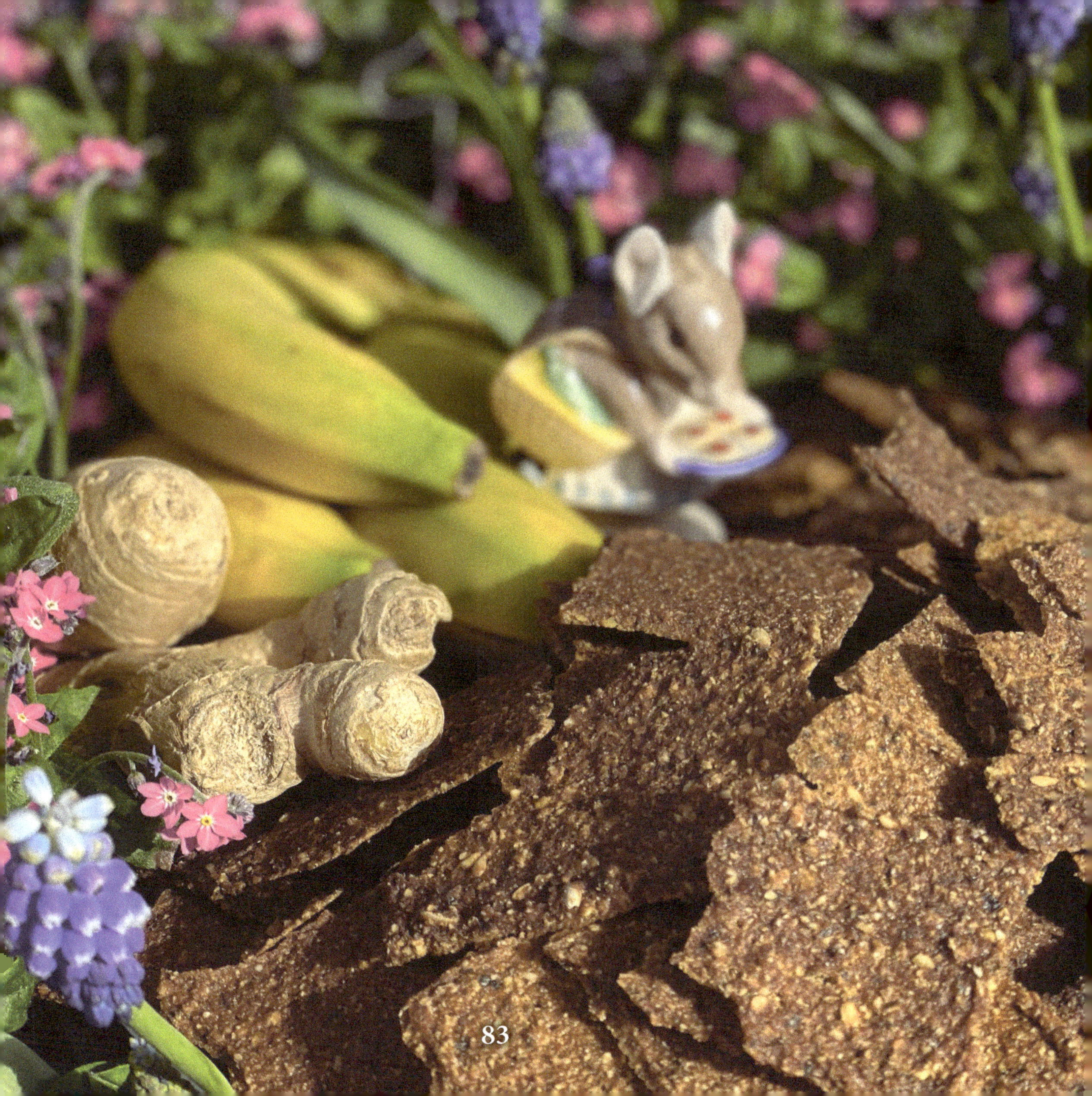

17

Cheeky Choco
PARSNIP PEANUT

The widely known chocolate bar which rhymes with "knickers", served as inspiration for this recipe.

The USDA lists the calorific value of a 2-ounce (57 gram) popular peanut/caramel/nougat bar as 280 kilocalories (1,200 kJ). That is approx. 20 percent of the daily energy needed by an average 7-year-old girl. Or equivalent to 24 medium-sized apples!

The list of ingredients mentioned on the packaging may go something like this: sugar, cocoa butter, chocolate, skimmed milk, lactose, milk fat, soy lecithin, artificial flavor, peanuts, corn syrup, sugar, palm oil, salt, egg whites, artificial flavor...

Ooof... I had no intention of using that many words for the intro... Nor would I place those listed ingredients in my blender or include them in my crackers.

What I really wanted to say here is simply: personally I LIKE PEANUTS.

I find the way these 'nuts' grow fascinating. Something like potatoes (peanuts are in the family of lentils and peas) – they grow and develop underground. I feel (and my body agrees) if the peanuts are grown and stored correctly, then they are just another wonderful gift from Mother Nature to add to our plate. Peanuts are nutritious legumes. (They contain some healthy fats, a combo of minerals vitamins, and fiber). What do YOU think?

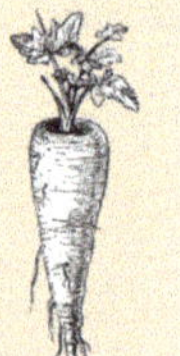

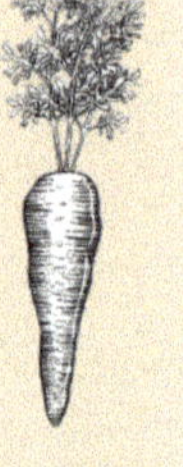

Ingredients:

3-5 parsnips

Carrot pulp from juicing (or a couple of whole carrots)

2-3 ripe bananas

1 level tablespoon of raw coconut oil

2-3 big cups of peanuts (buy them in a reputable health store in a raw state and then lightly roast them just before the cracker preparation begin)

Maca powder (approx. 3 heaped big spoons)

Dark unsweetened chocolate for a final drizzle

Optional:

Apples

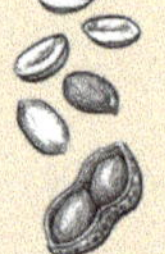

Process

Place the parsnips, carrot pulp, coconut oil, Maca powder, and a cup of water into a blender, and blend until the parsnips are chopped into very small bits. Add bananas and fresh, lightly roasted and cooled peanuts. Run the blender until the cracker mix looks almost smooth with some recognizable bits of nut remaining.

Spread the blended cracker mix evenly on the Teflex sheet placed on the dehydrator tray. Once spread evenly (think thin pizza crust) try to score the mix with the side of the spatula or blunt knife into slices or squares. If the consistency is still too runny – dehydrate it for a couple more hours and score it once the cracker mix thickens (meaning it's drier). Dry at 113 degrees F (45 degrees C) for approx. 5 hours. Check your crackers, flip them and peel off the sheets if possible. Peeling the crackers off sheets and leaving them on a bare mesh of dehydrator tray makes drying much faster – hence I try to peel the cracker mix from the sheets as soon as it's possible. Dehydrate for 4-5 hours more. Recheck the crackers and, if crispy-dry, store them in airtight boxes after a brief cooling down. If drying for a little longer is needed, you know what to do.

Maca powder adds that "caramel" hint to the nutty flavor of these crackers.

A handful of crackers makes everything better!

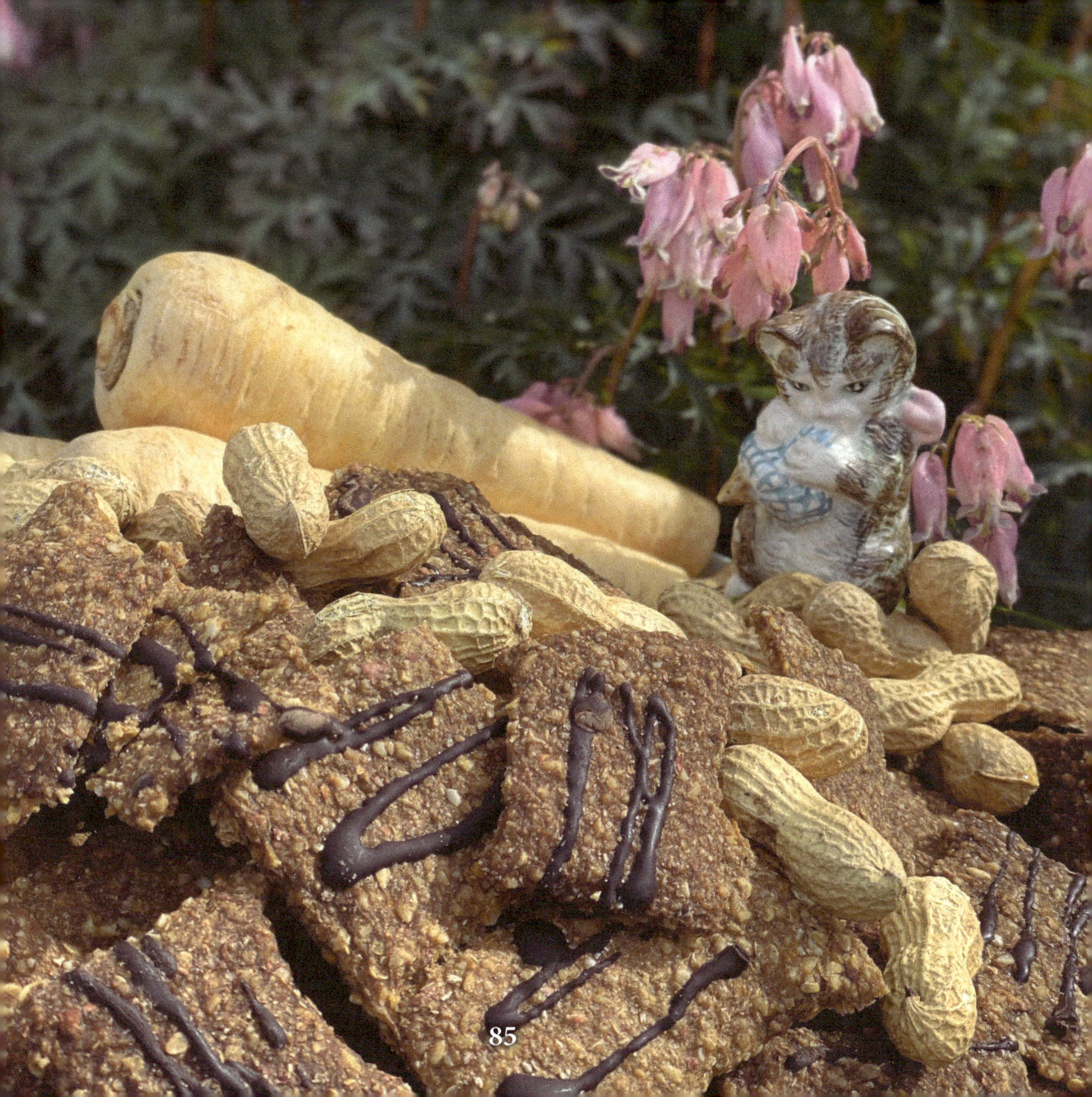

18

Crunchy cinnamony CARROTS with ALMOND flakes

Do you like fresh carrot juice?

I make mine in a centrifugal juicer from approx. 1 kg of carrots, 1-2 apples, and half a lemon. I also like to add ginger or turmeric. Drinking a glass of fresh carrot juice in the morning makes my body sing JOY.

Leftover apple/carrot pulp makes a great base for crackers in this recipe.

Spiced with cinnamon, which has a sweet, flavor-enhancing taste on its own, these crackers remind me of Christmas.

By the way — for this cracker recipe the blender is not necessary as the cracker mixture can be made with bare hands.

Ingredients:

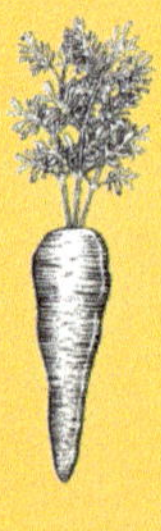
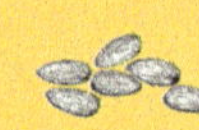
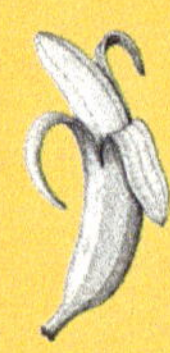

Carrot and apple pulp from juicing (if you're adding other ingredients to your carrot-apple-based juice, remember to remove the pure apple and carrot pulp you would like to use for crackers from the pulp collector – before it mixes/ is buried under other pulps). What I would do: First juice the carrot and apple – stop the juicer – empty the pulp collector – continue juicing the rest of the juice ingredients which are not meant for today's cracker recipe.

Raw almond flakes 300 g

Cinnamon powder

1 level tablespoon of raw coconut oil

Ripe banana (1-3: depends on how chewy and sweet you want the crackers to be – ripe bananas add these attributes.)

Optional:

Agave syrup and *raw shredded coconut*

Process

Feel free to add some parsnips into your carrot-apple juice, and therefore add parsnip pulp to the final crackers for extra mineral and fiber content.

Mix all the ingredients in the bowl (that's easily done with your hands) until the cinnamon and coconut oil are distributed evenly.

Place on a silicon sheet (which is placed on top of the dehydrator tray) in a thin layer, using just your hands or your favorite spatula. Place in the dehydrator, I set mine to 113° F and allow approximately eight hours of time. Dehydrate until you like the crunchiness.

In case you have a blender, here's a faster way to prepare this recipe: blend the bananas with the cinnamon, coconut oil and water. Pour the blended 'sauce' over the carrot/apple pulp from the juicer and add almond flakes. Finish mixing these ingredients by hand until the almond flakes are distributed evenly.

Carrot is rich in vitamins (vitamin A, provitamin beta carotene, alpha carotene, vitamin C, vitamin K), minerals (potassium, calcium), antioxidants such as lutein, zeaxanthin, lycopene in red and anthocyanin in purple carrots. Raw carrots are a wonderful low-calorie high-fiber food, with a low glycemic index.

Cinnamon is a multifaceted medicinal plant with several health benefits. Almost all its parts, such as the flower, leaf, bark, and root, have some culinary and medicinal use. However, its bark is used most extensively and is often associated with major health benefits (it contains antibacterial and antifungal properties.) Cinnamon is generally regarded as safe to give to kids in small sensible amounts. Luckily cinnamon doesn't commonly cause an allergic reaction in children or adults.

Cinnamon contains phytochemicals that boost the brain's ability to utilize glucose. Adequate and prolonged use of cinnamon might help boost cognitive development among children. The only true cinnamon is called Ceylon cinnamon, also known as cinnamommum verum or cinnamomum zeylanicum.

Tip: try to source and buy good quality cinnamon sticks and grind them at home.

These crackers aren't just for Christmas!

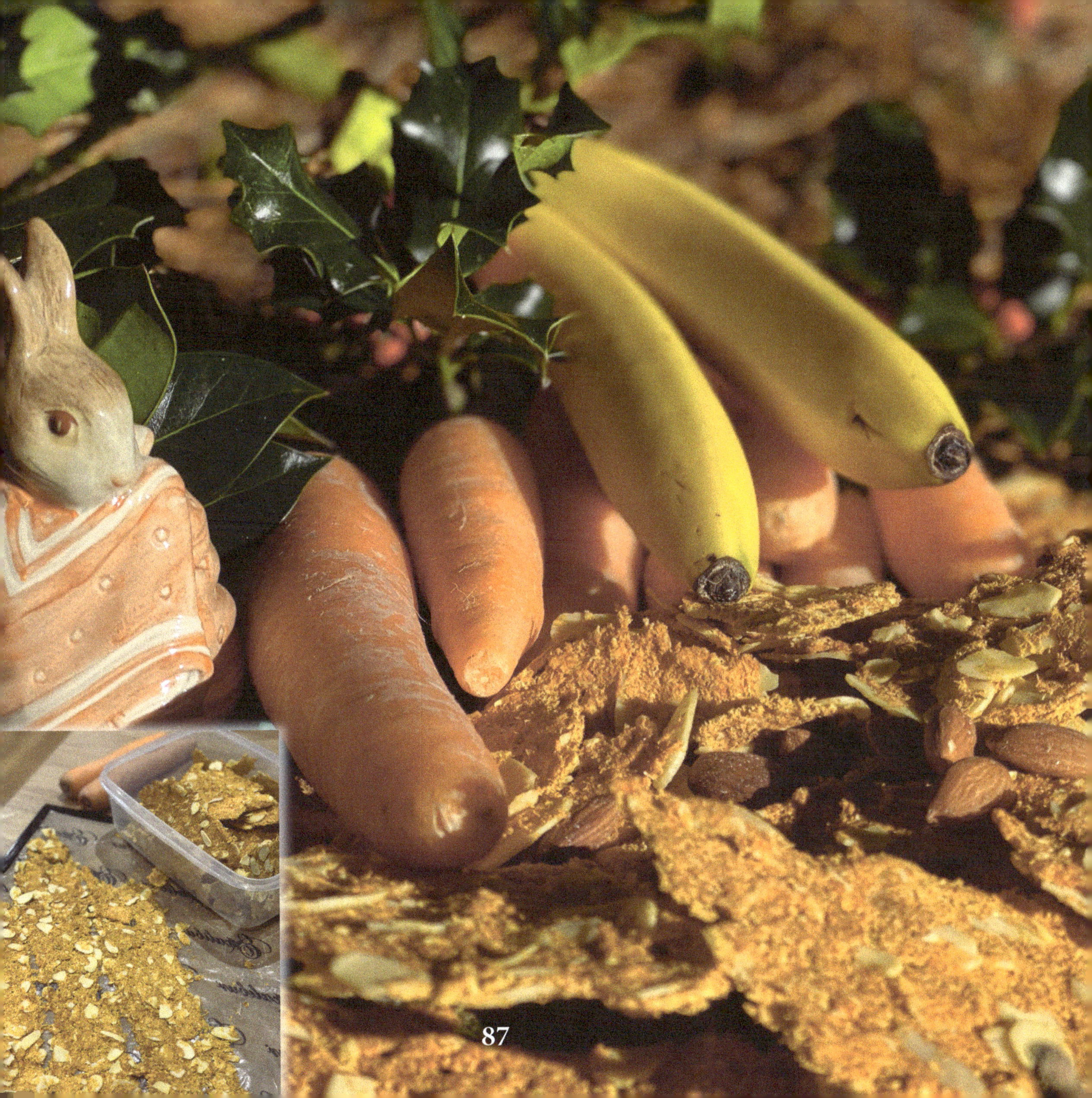

19

Jolly PEAR-STRAWBERRY-APPLE leathers

These fruit leathers are delicious!

Fruit leathers, also known as fruit strips or fruit roll-ups are healthy-sounding snacks. However, many fruit roll-ups sold in stores contain too much added sugar and possibly even artificial ingredients. If you are a parent, you have most likely come across these in conventional stores. You may even happen to have some in your kitchen cupboard on a snack-for-kids shelf. I challenge you now: put this book down and go read those labels. Most likely some of these products are fruit-flavored candy, not healthy snacks. Of course, fruit in its whole unprocessed form is the healthiest fruit snack we can eat. I consider the dried whole fruits the second best.

In case your kids are not the easiest to convince about grabbing fresh fruit every day, homemade fruit roll-ups can be a great option for them. To make these you can basically take any fruit you have lying around. Do you have a surplus of any fruits you or your neighbor or local farmer recently harvested?

Purée it and dehydrate it into a nutritious chewy high-energy snack. These will be your own. Free of sweeteners, colorants, and preservatives. Made at home with love.

You will want to select fruit that is ripe or even slightly overripe.

For my recipe I used:

Ingredients:

Organic ripe pears, apples and strawberries.

The ratio is totally up to you (I went 1:1:1).

Some days I juice apples and pears for a morning juice combo (I add veggies to my juice too, but remember to keep the fruit-only pulp separate from the veggie pulp, with the intention of making fruit leathers out of it. Store the veggie pulp for another time/recipe.)

Optional:

*Add **lemon juice** for an extra tangy flavor*

*Add **ripe mango/bananas** for extra 'chewiness'*

*Add **pumpkin/parsnip** if you wish to 'sneak' some veggies into your creation*

Process

If you would like to add some healthy raw seeds (healthy fats) then maybe opt for sunflower seeds, chia, or yellow flaxseed and blend until your kids can't detect them in the finished snack.

Blend all the ingredients in your blender, adding filtered water if needed. Spread the blended cracker mix evenly on the Teflex sheet in the dehydrator tray. Place in the dehydrator for a couple of hours at 113 degrees F (45 degrees C). Check up on your leathers: once they are dry enough and not 'runny' and sticky anymore — peel them of the silicone sheets.

Roll the leather into a tight tidy roll and with a sharp knife cut into the length of your choice.

Tips for more combos:

The possibilities of combinations are endless. Interesting ones can be rhubarb & strawberry, blueberry & chia, bananas, raspberry & peach.

You can partially dip in melted dark chocolate to add a festive/party twist to this jolly treat.

Dobrú chuť!

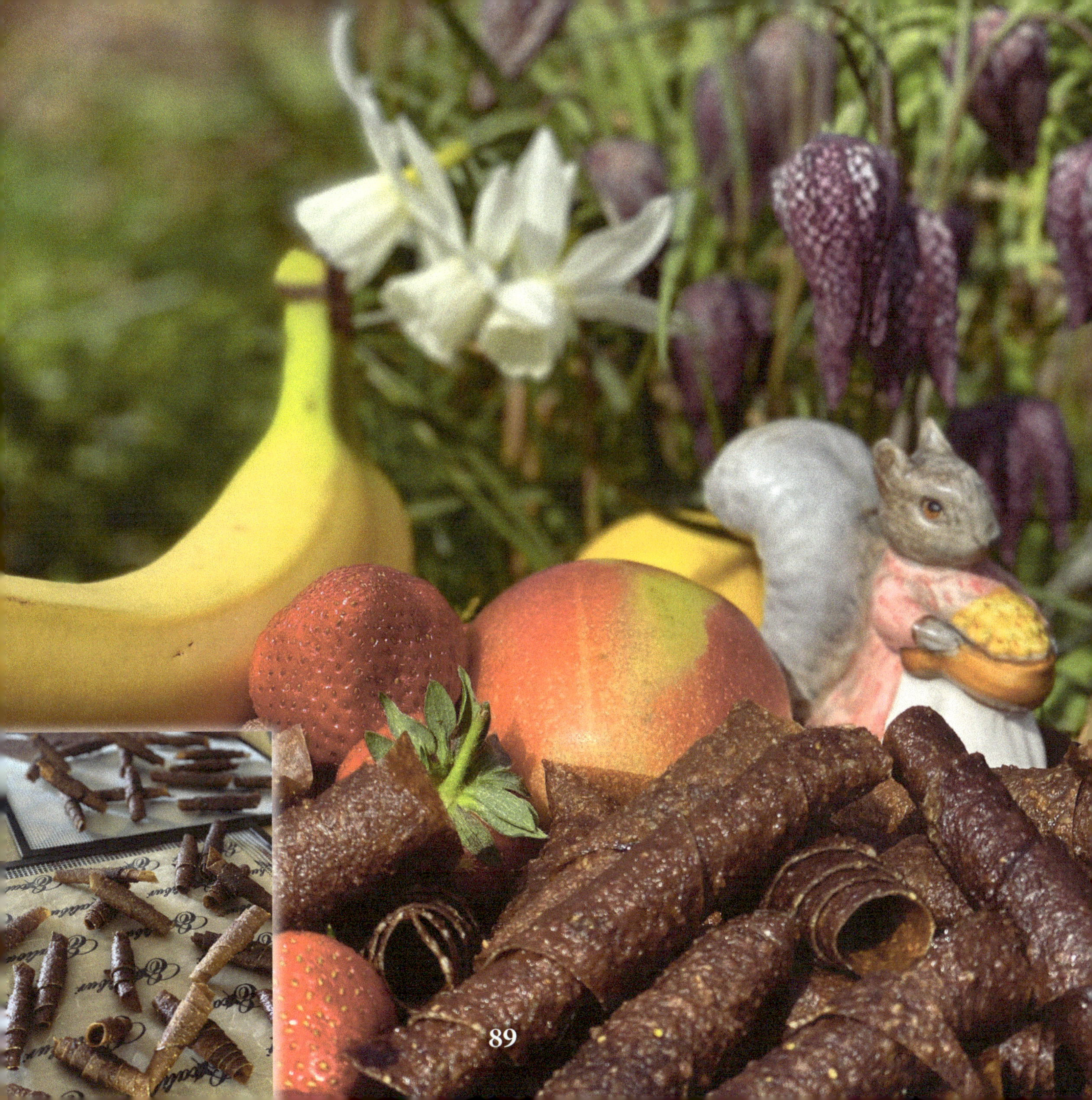

20

Mellow yellow MELON and ELDERFLOWER

Are you living in a part of the world where elderflowers blossom in spring? They are beautiful, aren't they? The whole elder plant has medicinal properties but it is mostly used as tinctures available in herbal stores. The flowers make wonderful aromatic slightly sweet and cooling diaphoretic tea. Try it on its own or add lemon, ginger and honey.

Elderflower can be very helpful when you or your kids have a cold or fever. Combine it with yarrow, peppermint, and catnip in a tea or infusion. This combo helps the body fight infections naturally, bringing on a sweat and helping overall relaxation. The flowers of the elder strengthen the upper respiratory tract and help remove phlegm. Do you suffer from pollen allergies? I believe even in a form as simple as my crackers, elderflower pollen can be helpful, especially if ingested daily for a couple of weeks before your seasonal allergies start — as a 'desensitizer' for the body. The flower infusion can be used as a gargle for sore throats, mouthwash for inflamed gums, or an eyewash for conjunctivitis, tired sore eyes, or twitching eyelids.

Elderflower tea with its inflammation-reducing effect can help with rheumatism, gout, and arthritis. It also has a diuretic effect which in consequence helps the body to relieve fluid retention and get rid of toxins. Elderflowers are the mildest and the safest part of the plant, even mild enough for small children to use. Its relaxant qualities help in the form of an evening tea, while infused drops induce peaceful sleep. It can be helpful for relieving bronchospasms for asthma sufferers, can soothe nerves, allay anxiety, and lift depression.

I challenge you here dear readers — because elderflowers make an excellent spring tonic and blood purifier- let's try to take a cup every morning before breakfast for a few weeks in spring and experience new energy and a restoration of health with a new power. And once you are on it, harvest baskets of these beautiful fragrant cream color flowers for this cracker recipe.

Ingredients:

1 ripe yellow gala melon (cantaloupe or honeydew are great alternatives)

A big bowl of fresh elderflowers

2-4 ripe bananas

Half of the peeled lemon without seeds

2 cups of raw sesame seeds

1 level tablespoon of raw coconut oil

Optional:

*Ripe **pineapple, parsnip, raw local honey, papaya, peach***

Process

Clean the melon, peel the skin, and remove the seeds. To prepare the flowers, which are hopefully harvested from clean, wild places far from roads, I normally do not wash them in order to preserve all the pollen. Just cut off the green stalks. Place all the ingredients in the blender, add a little bit of water if needed and blend until you are happy with the texture.

If you like the texture of whole sesame seeds in your crackers, add them to blend only at the end. So yes, honey, chia seeds, pineapple, papaya, peach, or parsnip are optional and can help to create new, interesting variations of this healing cracker recipe.

Tip: remember to dry loads of extra elderflowers for the months to come. Store them in glass airtight containers in a dark cupboard to use in a tea infusion or in this recipe for times when fresh blossom is not in reach.

Other things one can try and create from elderflower are elderflower champagne, syrup, or vinegar... for more recipes and ideas visit my blog www.23blossom.com

Continue with the METHOD on pages 40-41

Cup of tea and cracker anyone?

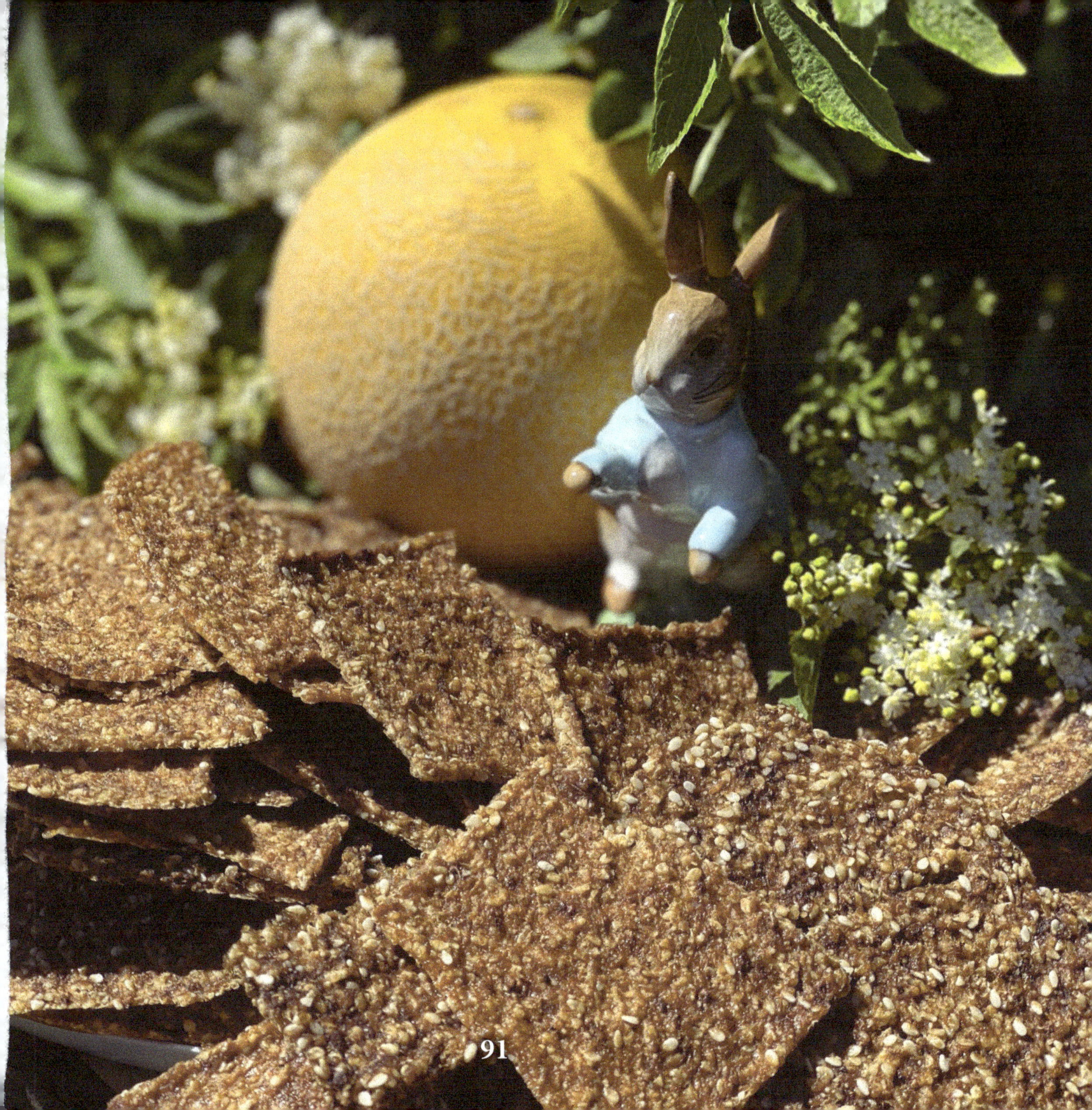

21

Healing DANDELION HONEY LEMON

I absolutely love these crackers. These crackers have the potential to become yummy overloads to the senses, especially if you have access to local high-quality honey. Close your eyes and smell them. Amazing. And you and your family are about to get a huge hit of healing power!

Yes, I'm talking about those yellow flowers, many refer to as 'just weeds'. Dandelion is an absolute superfood, a natural medicine to me. It is a gift from nature. A great source of antioxidants and vitamin A and E which prevent free radical damage, B complex, vitamins C and D, calcium, iron, manganese, magnesium, phosphorus, potassium, sodium, phytoestrogens, and saponins. Dandelions are great for your colon and its flora, help with liver & digestion, kidneys, blood & circulation... the list is very long, there would be no space left for the recipe here if I kept going. Once again read the blog post on www.23blossom.com if you care to learn more.

Ingredients:

Bowl of fresh dandelion flowers

Approx. 150 ml of honey

1-2 lemons

3 parsnips

1 medium pineapple

2-4 ripe bananas

1-2 cups sunflower seeds

1 level tablespoon of raw coconut oil

Optional:

1-3 apples

Process

For the crackers: I use only the yellow petals of dandelion flowers, as the green stalks and leaves taste bitter. (In our kitchen there is lots of use for the green bits of this plant too, but not in this cracker recipe which is designed to be liked by kids.) For one batch of crackers go for as big a bowl of yellow petals as you can get, or as many flowers as you and your kids have the patience to collect and 'unstalk'.

I normally go out into clean nature on a sunny day when they blossom, collect a full basket of flowers and then sit somewhere nice and cut the yellow bits from the green part of each flower, either with scissors or a sharp knife on the chopping board. Another way to do it: go out on a flower hunt with scissors and cut the yellow petals directly into a clean Tupperware or a clean paper bag. I do not wash the flowers as I want to preserve as much pollen on them as possible. Hence, to be safe, I always collect flowers from gardens or places far from roads, where I can be sure no chemicals have been sprayed. I think it is important to make the crackers the same day the petals are collected. (Though it's fine to store them in the fridge until the next day, if you must. I like to imagine there is still some SUN in them when I get them home and play with the cracker mix so I try to make them ASAP.) Peel the lemons, cut in half and remove their seeds. Place them in a blender with the parsnips, pineapple chunks, honey, coconut oil, and approx. half a cup of warm water. Blend until the parsnip is homogenized into small bits. Add more water if necessary.

After that, add the bananas, seeds, and dandelion petals. Blend until you like the structure of the mix. I personally like to see some yellow petals in my crackers as a sunny reminder, so I keep half of the petals and add to the blender at the end. This way they do not disappear in the blending.

Continue with the METHOD on pages 40-41

Crackers don't give you love handles!

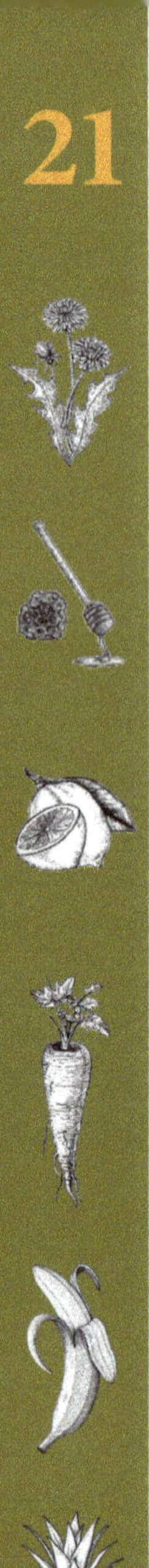

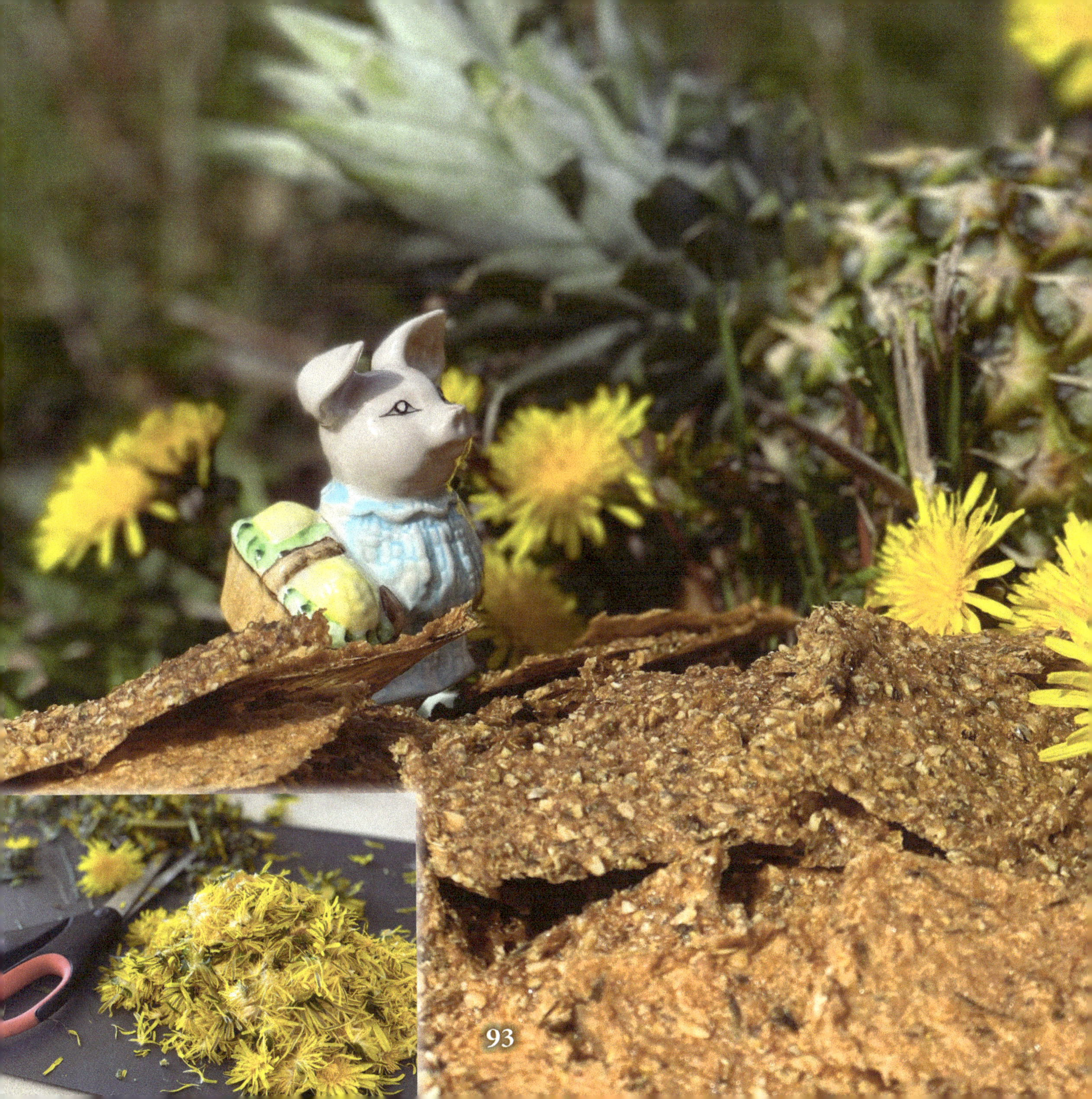

22

Awesome APRICOT

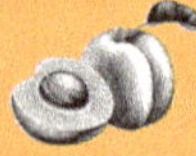

Are apricots healthy for kids? Yes! Like all orange-colored fruits and vegetables, apricots contain carotenoids, which the body converts to vitamin A, which supports healthy eyes, immunity, and skin... There is fiber, lots of potassium, and an abundance of vitamins in this pleasant cousin of the peach. There is really no reason for not adding apricots to a daily fruit plate selection for you and your kids, especially when apricots are in season. I have three majestic apricot trees in my garden, so I choose to preserve them in the form of yummy apricot crackers when the harvest is abundant.

Ingredients:

2 kg of ripe apricots

3 parsnips

2 carrots

1 level tablespoon of raw coconut oil

300 g of raw seeds of your choice (I like the mix of hemp seed, sesame, sunflower, chia)

Optional:

*Add ripe **orange or banana***
Juice from ½ lemon

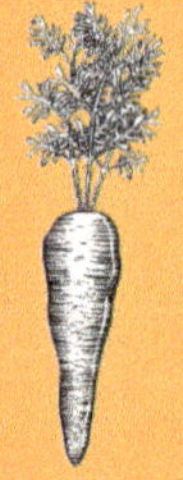

Process

Halve the washed apricots and remove the stones.

In case no fresh ripe apricots are available, you can improvise and use dried apricots instead. In that case, make sure you soak them for a couple of hours, and rinse well afterward. Please don't use the soaking water.

(Dried apricots are widely available in stores and are treated with sulfur dioxide (E220), their color, as a result, is vivid orange. Organic fruit not treated with sulfur vapor is darker in color and has a coarser texture. Generally, the lighter the color, the higher the SO2 content. The main point of soaking and rinsing is to remove the SO2 residues.)

Add all the ingredients to the blender together with up to a cup of warm filtered water.

Blend until you like the consistency of the blend.

Spread the blended cracker mix evenly on the Teflex sheet placed on the dehydrator tray. Once spread evenly (think thin pizza crust) try to score the mix with the side of the spatula or blunt knife into slices or squares. If the consistency is still too runny – dehydrate it for a couple more hours and score it once the cracker mix thickens (meaning it's drier). Dry at 113 degrees F (45 degrees C) for approx. 5 hours. Check your crackers, flip them and peel off the sheets if possible. Peeling the crackers off sheets and leaving them on a bare mesh of dehydrator tray makes drying much faster – hence I try to peel the cracker mix from the sheets as soon as it's possible. Dehydrate for 4-5 hours more. Recheck the crackers and, if crispy-dry, store them in airtight boxes after a brief cooling down. If drying for a little longer is needed, you know what to do.

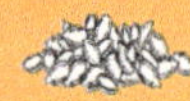

Bon appetit!

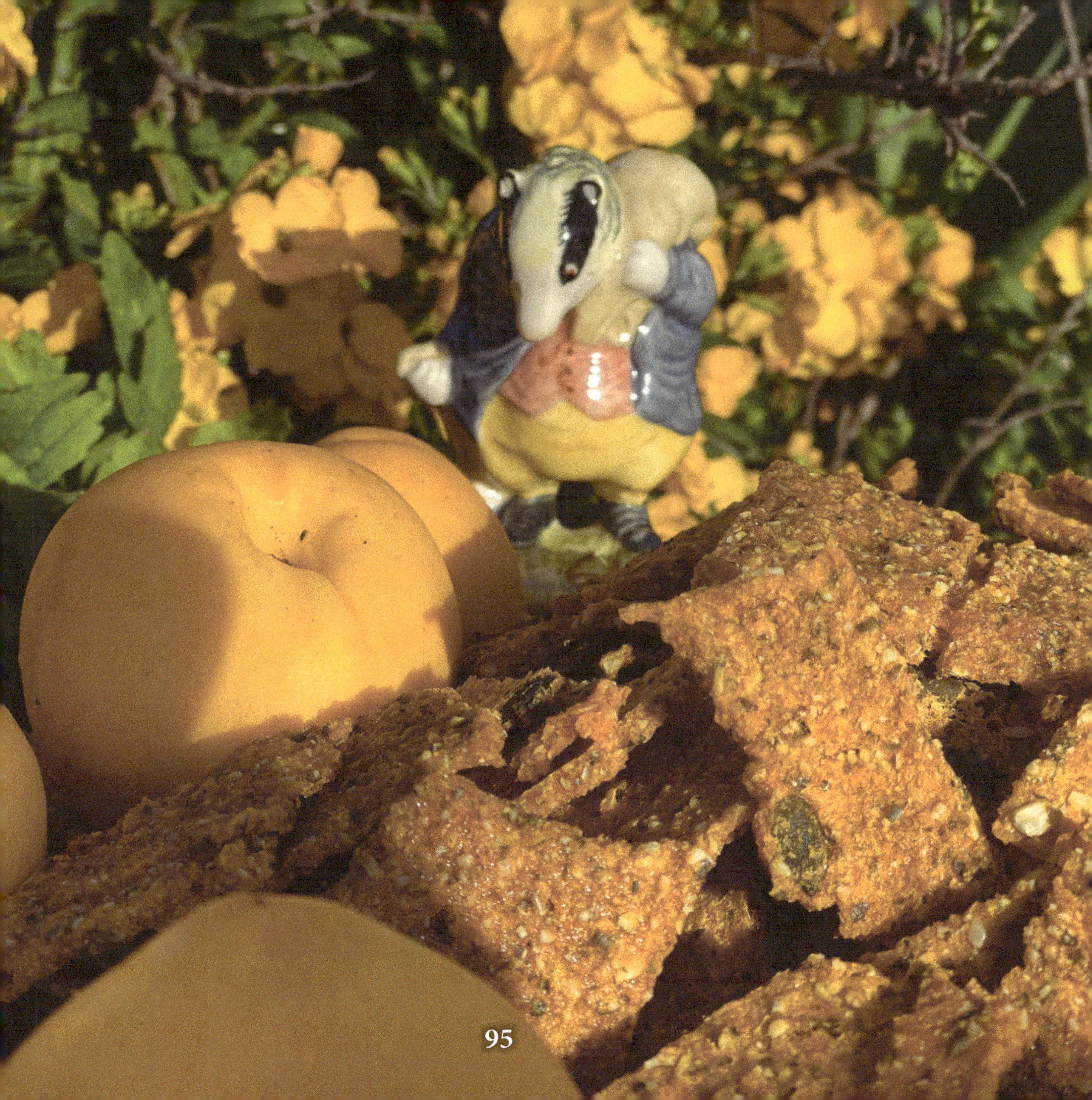

23

Adorable sliced APPLES with CINNAMON and almond flakes

This recipe is super simple and loved by many... This could be one of the first recipes I recommend you try from this entire book. (A good one to test your new, or newly rediscovered, dehydrator with.) If you want to impress your guests, or ever feel like convincing someone to start a dehydrating journey of their own, I would bet on this one. Crunchiness is a universal language!

Ingredients:

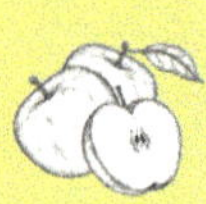

Raw almond flakes. (The amount of flakes you use really depends on you and your naughty "nut tooth" and obviously on the number of apples you're about to turn into crunchy slices. The amount I normally use is approx. 100 g almond flakes to 1 kg of apples.)

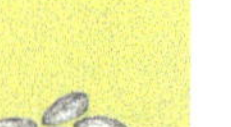

Apples (any type really. I like to experiment and try different varieties of apples. The difference in outcome may be subtle, but still exciting for apple lovers like me.)

Ingredients for 'sauce':

1 very ripe banana

1 carrot

1 heaped tablespoon of raw coconut oil

Cinnamon (up to your preference how much you use — I normally use roughly 1 tablespoon to 1kg of apples)

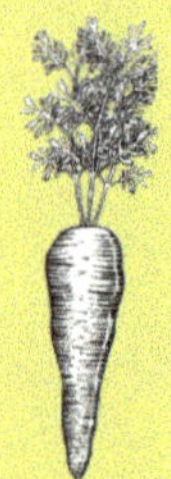

Cup of filtered water

Process

Yesss, a very observant reader may have noticed here — these are very similar ingredients to those for recipe 18. Yet… get ready to have a totally different, flawless experience when tasting these. This is another recipe where we do not need a big blender. A small blender is sufficient for preparing the 'sauce' for coating the sliced apples. Let's begin by slicing the apples.

Truly there's nothing better, faster, or more efficient I know of in the kitchen for slicing your apples than a mandoline food slicer. I highly recommend them, but before going any further with this recipe I need to warn you: PLEASE, do use this type of slicer with due care and diligence! Give it the respect it deserves, wear a protective glove, and always always always use the slicing guard/food holder... I will not say more, most probably I'll write a whole blog post about safety and the way to use and clean (yes, cleaning may be even more dangerous than using) these slicers: check www.23blossom.com.

And no, you don't need a slicer, you can simply cut your apples into thin (approx. 3-4 mm) even slices. Did you slice all the apples? Place them in a very big bowl. Then to prepare the sauce to coat the 'apple slithers' as my husband likes to call them:

Place the banana, carrot, coconut oil, cinnamon, and water into the blender, and blend until totally smooth. Pour the brown cinnamon flavored sauce over the apple slithers in a bowl. Add the raw almond flakes. Now the real fun begins – I normally use my hands – massage the sauce all over the apple slices, and aim to distribute the almond flakes evenly. Place the apple slices on silicone dehydrator sheets in a single layer, preferably not overlapping each other.

(continue to the next page...)

Crunch above the rest!

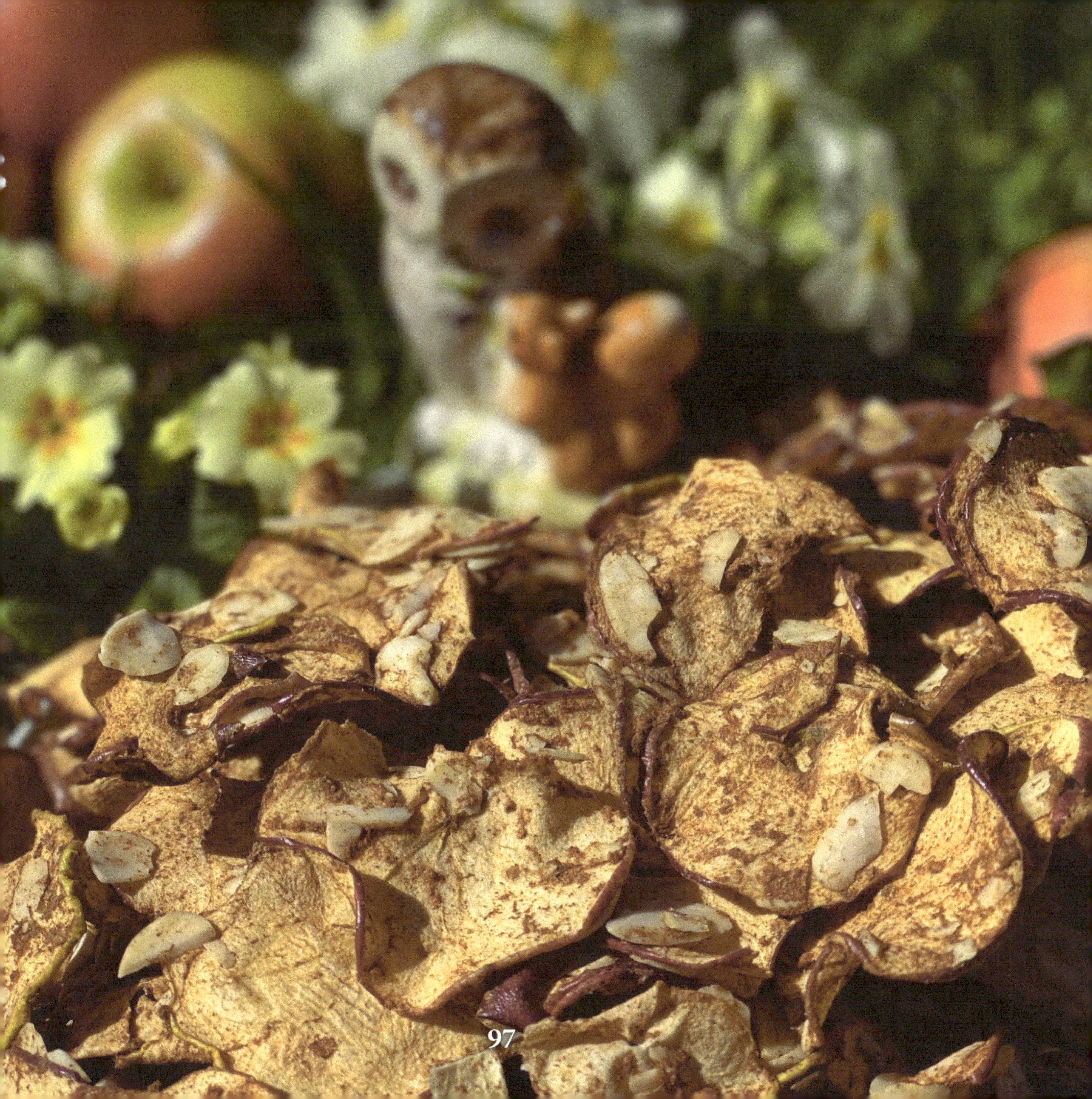

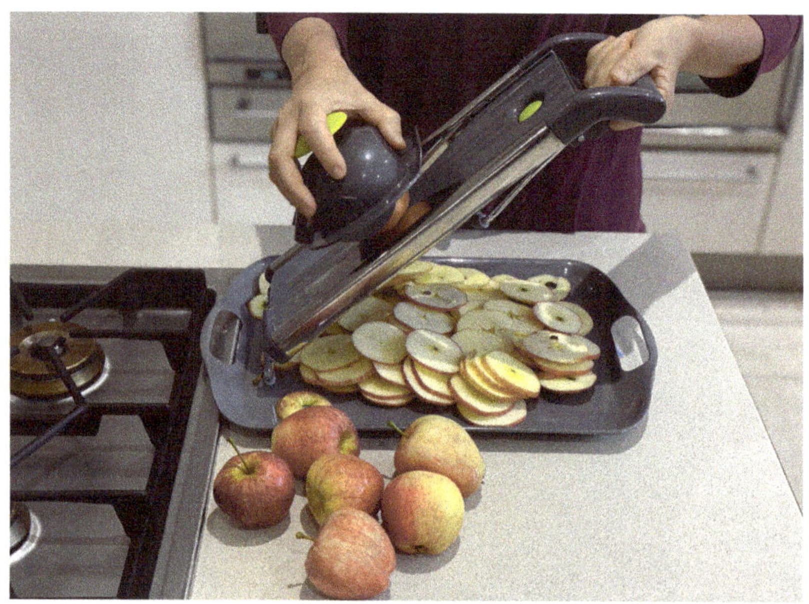 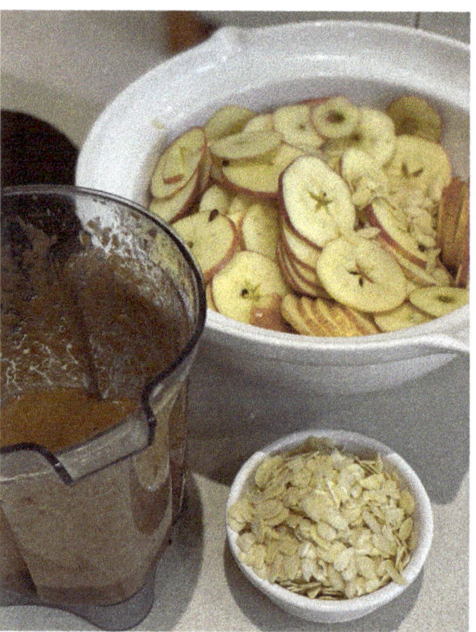

To me, it feels like meditation – sitting cross-legged on top of our polished kitchen top listening to music and placing apple slice after apple slice on a silicone sheet, in rows like my little Cinnamon Army. Once all done, place in the dehydrator. I set mine on 113°F and allow approximately eight hours of time. Dehydrate until totally crispy. Once possible, maybe halfway through the dehydrating time, peel the apple slices from the silicone sheet and continue dehydrating directly on the bare mesh.

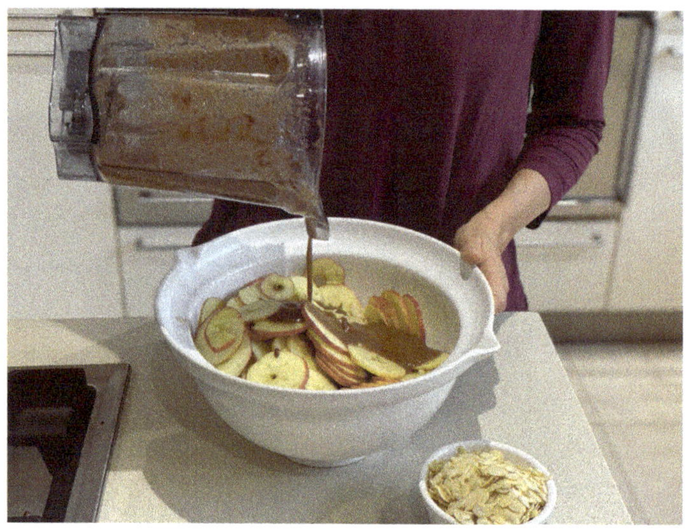 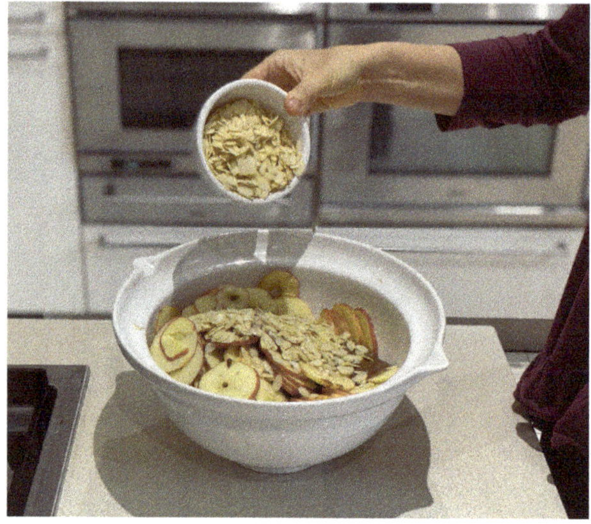

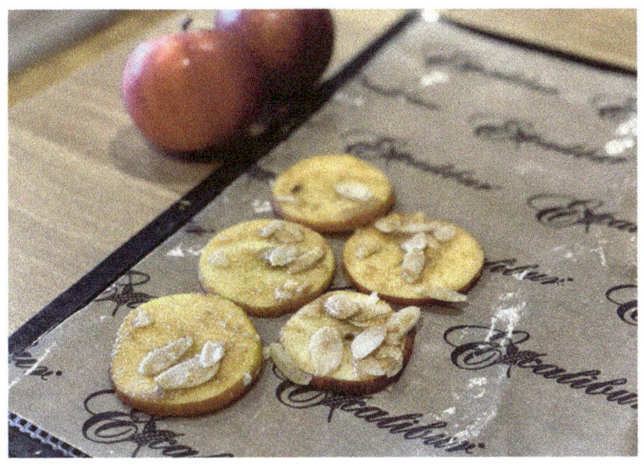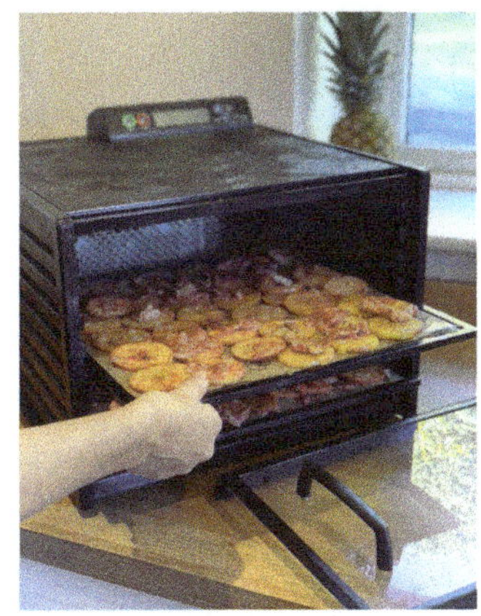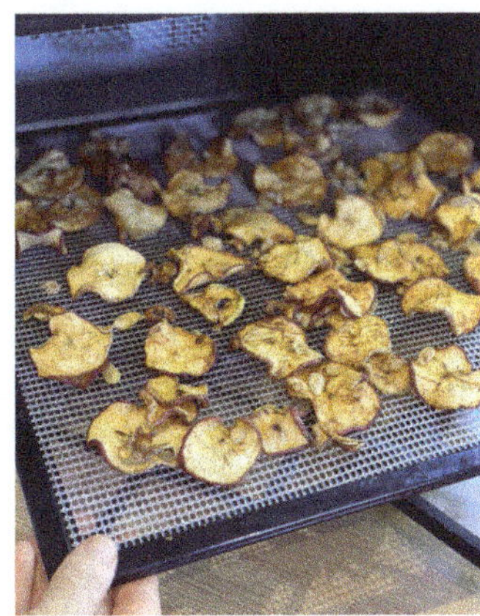

Alternative sauces *for coating your apple slices:*

1. ripe banana + 1 parsnip + heaped kitchen spoon of coconut oil + heaped kitchen spoon of cinnamon powder + 1 cup of fresh or frozen raspberries + cup of almond flakes (although add the flakes after the blending)

2. ripe banana + small spoon of coconut oil + 1 cup of raw pumpkin seeds + ½ cup of chia seeds + heaped kitchen spoon of cinnamon powder

3. big ripe mango peeled + cup of ripe fresh or frozen strawberries + cup of chia seeds + dash of lemon juice + heaped kitchen spoon of coconut oil

Preparation in each of these sauce options is the same: blend all the ingredients with a cup of warm filtered water.

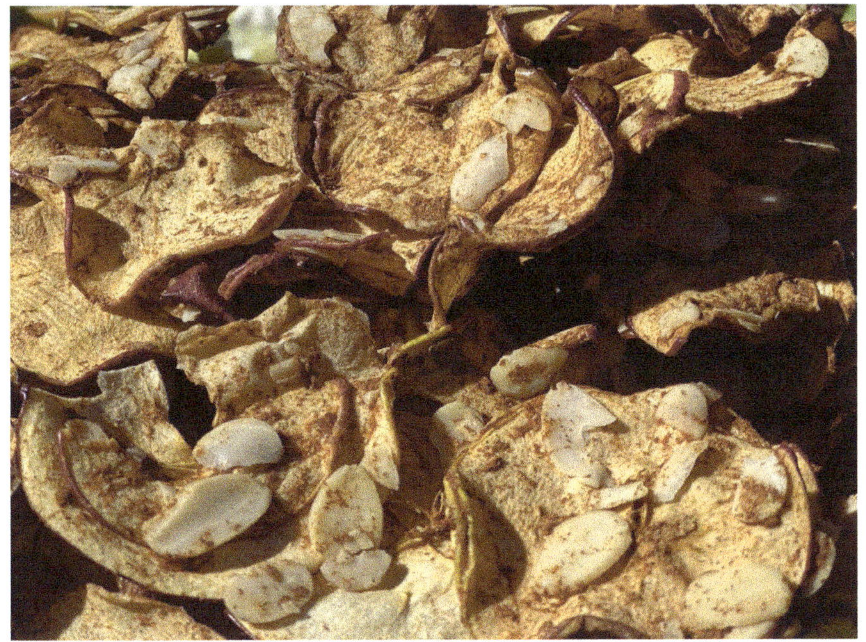

Tip 1: Try to add the berries to the sauce only once everything else is blended smooth, and whizz only briefly – so the nice bits of berries still remain to be seen once the dehydrated treat is done and ready to eat.

Tip 2: Experiment with different amounts of sauce! I learned that I prefer to have double the amount of sauce! I love my apple slices totally and abundantly covered/coated – as the coating itself is so yummy especially, when the cracker is fully dehydrated.

24

Cracking GREEN APPLES
with pumpkin seeds

Maybe the last time you saw them was in the gym, or sitting in a lovely hotel reception bowl? Hmm, maybe later. Thank you… If you're not one of those green apple lovers, I challenge you here: GIVE GREEN APPLES a chance! To try this cracking cocoa powder dusted delicacy we need…

Ingredients:

Green apples

Raw pumpkin seeds, slightly crushed

1 heaped tablespoon of raw coconut oil

Cocoa powder (preferably unsweetened)

Agave syrup (to sweeten this treat if you wish)

Agave syrup together with coconut oil will help to bind the seeds to apple slices.

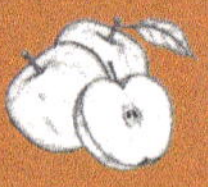

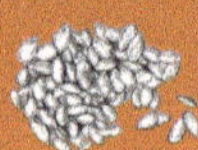

Process

Wash the apples.

Slice them all with a mandolin slicer into a big bowl (experiment with the thickness of slices, I sliced these very thin. That's the way we like them. WARNING: Please note my comments about mandolin safety in recipe 23.) Add cocoa powder, coconut oil, pumpkin seeds, and agave syrup.

'Massage' all very well together with your hands, until the oil and cocoa are distributed evenly. Alternatively you can blend ½ cup of warm water with cocoa, agave syrup & a spoonful of coconut oil, and coat the apple slices with this 'sauce' with the pumpkin seeds sprinkled over the top.

Place on dehydrator trays in thin layers. Place in the dehydrator. I usually set mine at 113°F temperature and for approx. 8 hours. Keep tasting them, check if they are crunchy enough… Store in the fridge in an airtight container.

Green apples are packed with fiber, most notably one called PECTIN. In human digestion, pectin binds to cholesterol in the gastrointestinal tract and slows glucose absorption by trapping carbohydrates. Pectin is, therefore, a soluble dietary fiber, and also serves as a prebiotic to promote the growth of healthy bacteria in your gut. It also seems to help lower LDL cholesterol (as the increase in viscosity in the intestinal tract leads to reduced absorption of cholesterol from bile or food.) There are a number of minerals – iron, zinc, copper, manganese, potassium, a trace of calcium, vitamin A, B, C, K in green apples too.

Pumpkin seeds have an exceptional number of vitamins and minerals, which are essential for your kids' growth and development, like vitamin K, copper, iron, and magnesium. Pumpkin seeds are rich in protein and omega-3-fatty acids.

They are also one of the richest plant sources of zinc. Zinc is vital for normal growth and development of the reproductive organs and brain, and plays a role in the optimal functioning of the immune system, and much more. The deficiency of zinc in a kid's diet has been linked to increased colds and infections, impaired memory, decreased growth, learning disabilities, reduced attention span…

PS: I have to warn you – cocoa-dusted dried green apples are a bit of a messy snack if handled by little kids. For a less messy sliced apple snack option check the recipe 23 where I offer ideas for different 'apple coating sauces.' Another beautiful cracking sliced apples variation of this recipe is red apples with raw or lightly roasted hazelnut bits and cocoa. Simply replace green apples with red apples, and pumpkin seeds with hazelnuts and follow the exact same recipe and steps in preparation.

It's crunch o'clock!

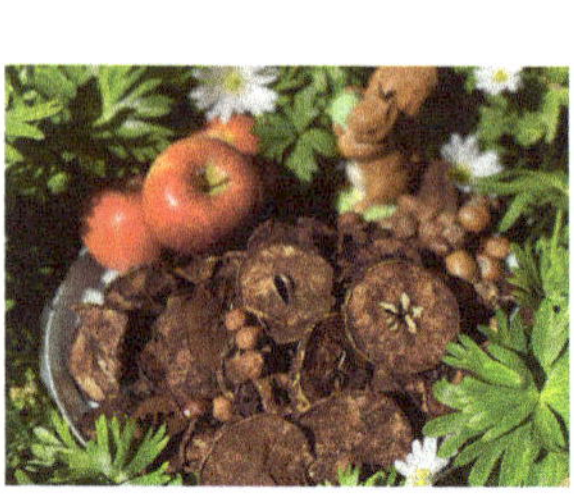

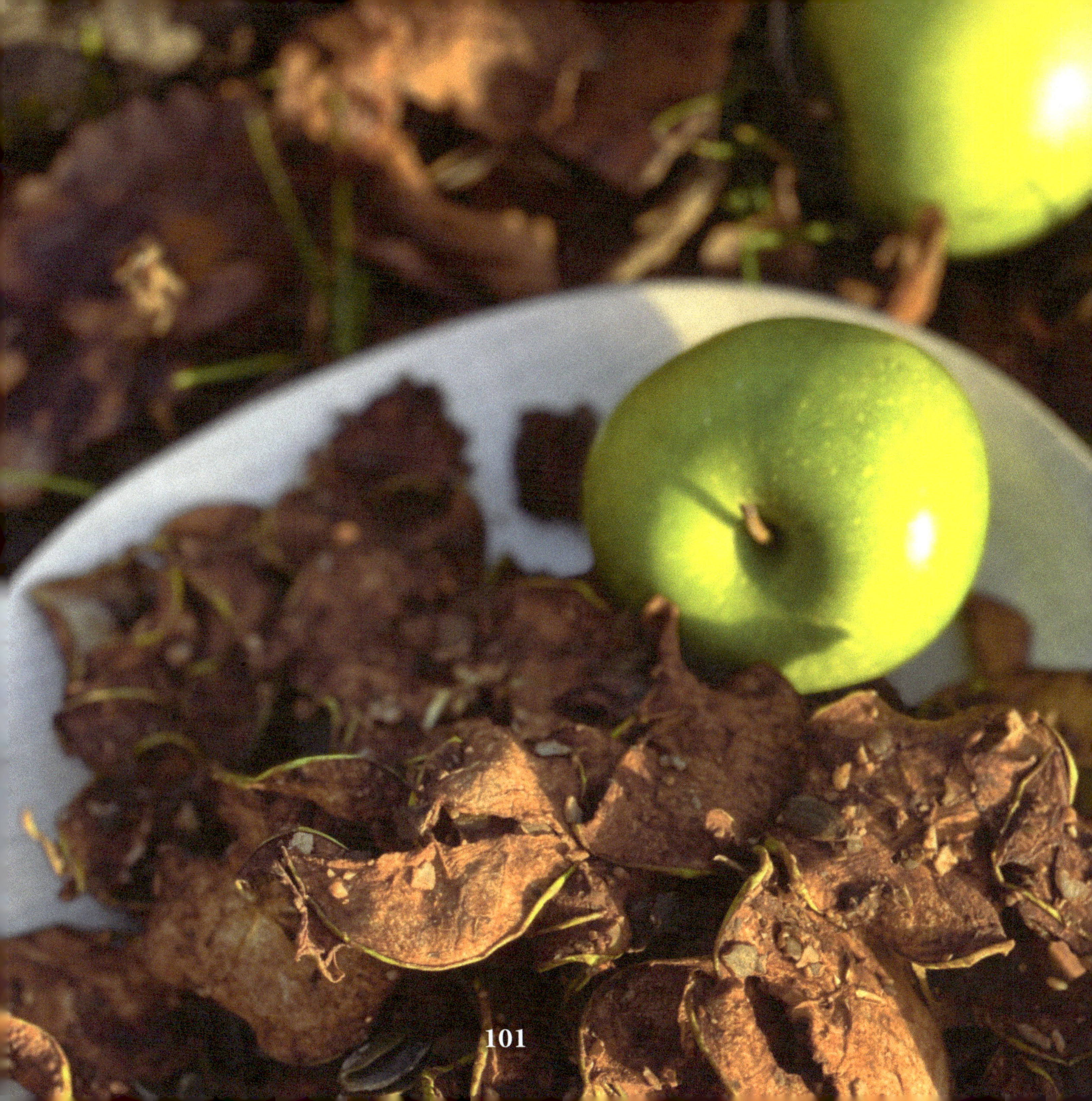

25

Krispy Krunchy KALE
krisps with sesame seeds

Before we proceed to some savory cracker recipes — it is time to share with you a super-easy-to-make green and yummy snack for the whole family. It is not a cracker, but pretty crispy regardless. This kale leaves/seeds/yeast combo has amazing nutritional value.

Ingredients:

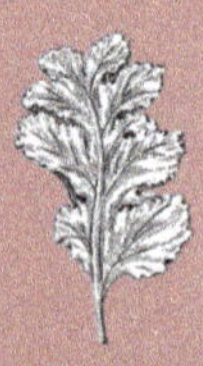

Fresh kale leaves (any type of kale will do)

Yeast flakes (search online or in your local supermarket or health store — these days they are not so hard to find)

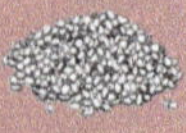

Raw sesame seeds (white or black, no preference)

A heaped tablespoon of coconut oil

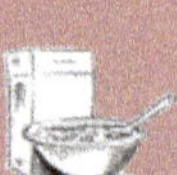

Process

Rip the kale off the stalks. Try to leave the leaf as a whole as possible. (I usually save the kale stalks for later and use them in savory veg crackers or blended veg soup.)

Massage the coconut oil into the kale and sprinkle generously with sesame seeds and yeast flakes.

Place on dehydrator sheets and dehydrate at 113°F degrees until thoroughly dry. *You can use your oven at a very low temperature.

Store in an airtight container in a cool dry place for up to 1 month. I bet there's no storing required as they get eaten fast…

Enjoy!

PS: You may want to consume these in moderation if you're a breastfeeding mother. Watch out and observe the baby, there is a chance it will get gassy. Kale belongs to the "brassica" family…

PPS: If you have more time on your hands — instead of coating the kale leaves just with coconut oil and sesame seeds, you could test 'cheesier' tastes and more filling variations of these crackers by doing the following. Soak ½ cup of raw cashew nuts for approx. six hours and, after rinsing them thoroughly, place in a blender together with one cup of yeast flakes, lemon juice from half a lemon, one parsnip and a small spoon of coconut oil. And 150 ml of warm water. Blend all these until totally smooth. Use this blend to 'coat' the kale leaves. Place the blended cashew nut coating sauce into a big bowl together with kale leaf chunks and sesame seeds. Use your hands to 'massage' the leaves to cover them all evenly.

Only then place the leaves in silicone sheets, and into the dehydrator.

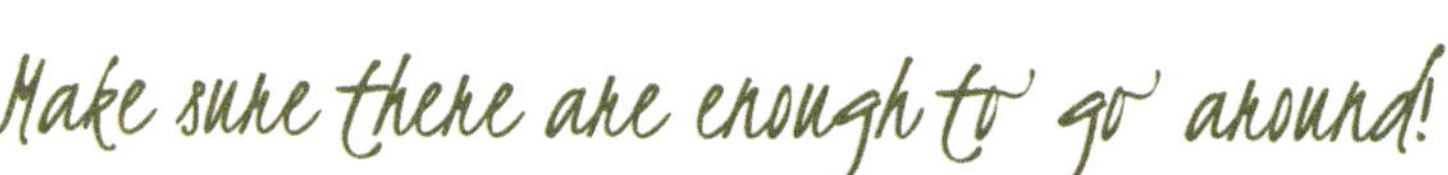

Make sure there are enough to go around!

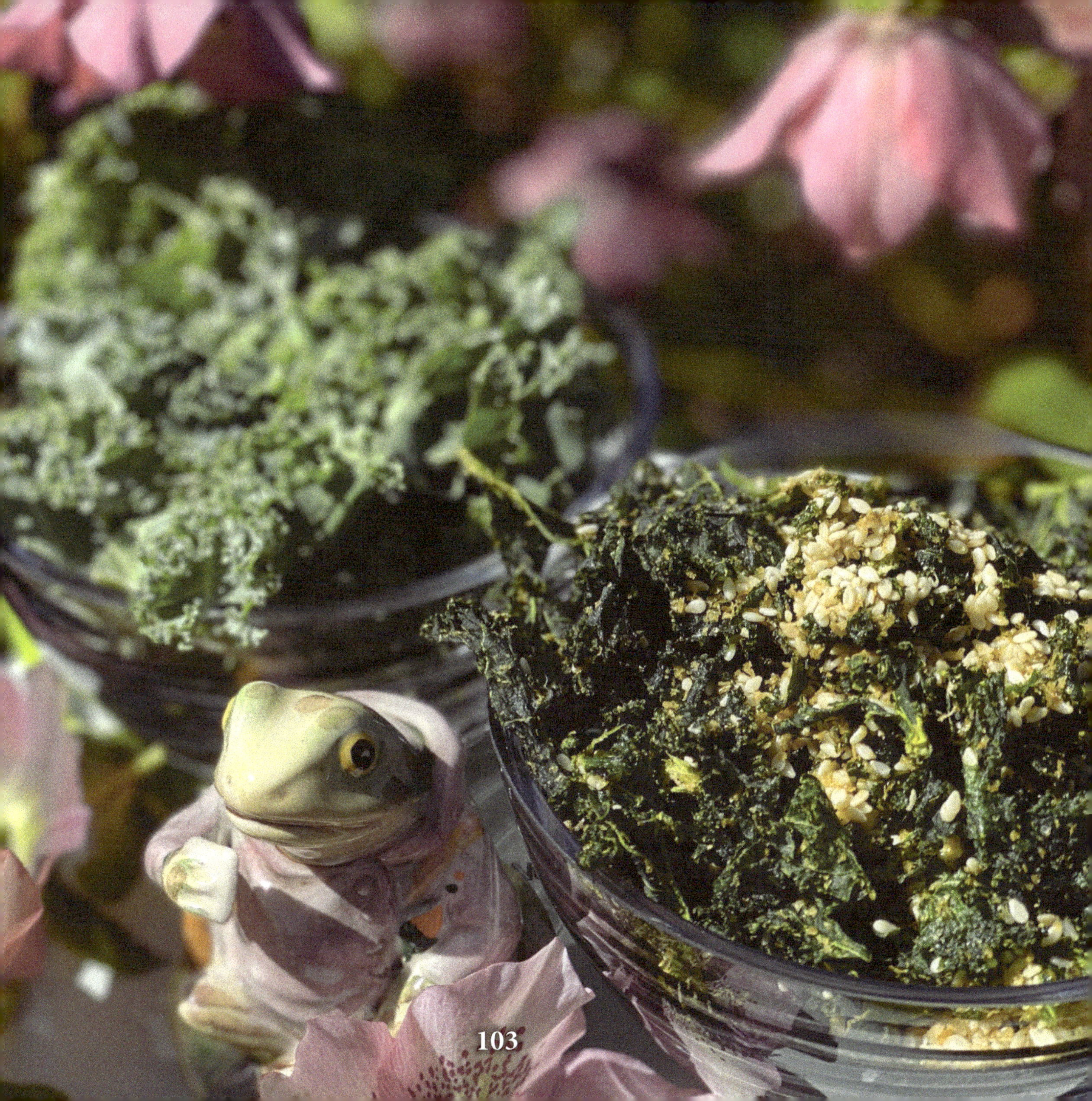

26

Blissful BASIL and TOMATO

Like apples, tomatoes also have the power to keep the doctor away. Especially the heart doctor it seems.

In French, tomatoes can be referred to as "pomme d'amour" aka LOVE APPLE and in the Czech language "rajské jablíčko" aka PARADISE APPLE. The wonderful power of words!

I love to wander in farmers' markets and admire tomatoes of all sizes colors and shapes.

I would urge you to show your children all these beautiful varieties and let them taste and express their personal opinions and preference. The interest and engagement in veggies, plants, and nature in general, can be nurtured from a very young age.

The main ingredients in this cracker recipe, tomatoes, and basil, are both easy to grow as pot plants even if you don't have a garden. Tomatoes are rich in antioxidants, vitamins A and C, folic acid, beta carotene, lycopene… Basil, apart from being super-rich in vitamin K, contains some minerals (copper, calcium, iron, manganese) vitamin C, and carotenoids as well essential oils with antibacterial effects.

It is a simple recipe.

Let me know how you liked it.

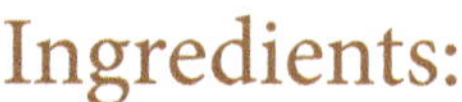

Ingredients:

1-2 kg tomato

Lots of fresh basil leaves (Approx. 3 big handfuls)

3-5 parsnips

1 level tablespoon of raw coconut oil

300 g of raw sunflower seeds (or mixed raw seeds of your choice)

Pinch of sea salt

Optional:

*I like to add some **brown flax seeds** for a more 'bread-like' feel*

*As well as: **sprouted pulses or grains** for more filling and vitamin B rich crackers*

Process

Place all the ingredients in a blender together with a cup of filtered water. Blend until you like the texture of the cracker mix.

Spread the blended cracker mix evenly on the Teflex sheet placed on the dehydrator tray. Once spread evenly (think thin pizza crust) try to score the mix with the side of the spatula or blunt knife into slices or squares. If the consistency is still too runny – dehydrate it for a couple more hours and score it once the cracker mix thickens (meaning it's drier). Dry at 113 degrees F (45 degrees C) for approx. 5 hours. Check your crackers, flip them and peel off the sheets if possible. Peeling the crackers off sheets and leaving them on a bare mesh of dehydrator tray makes drying much faster – hence I try to peel the cracker mix from the sheets as soon as it's possible. Dehydrate for 4-5 hours more. Recheck the crackers and, if crispy-dry, store them in airtight boxes after a brief cooling down. If drying for a little longer is needed, you know what to do.

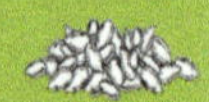

Oh, what a cracker!

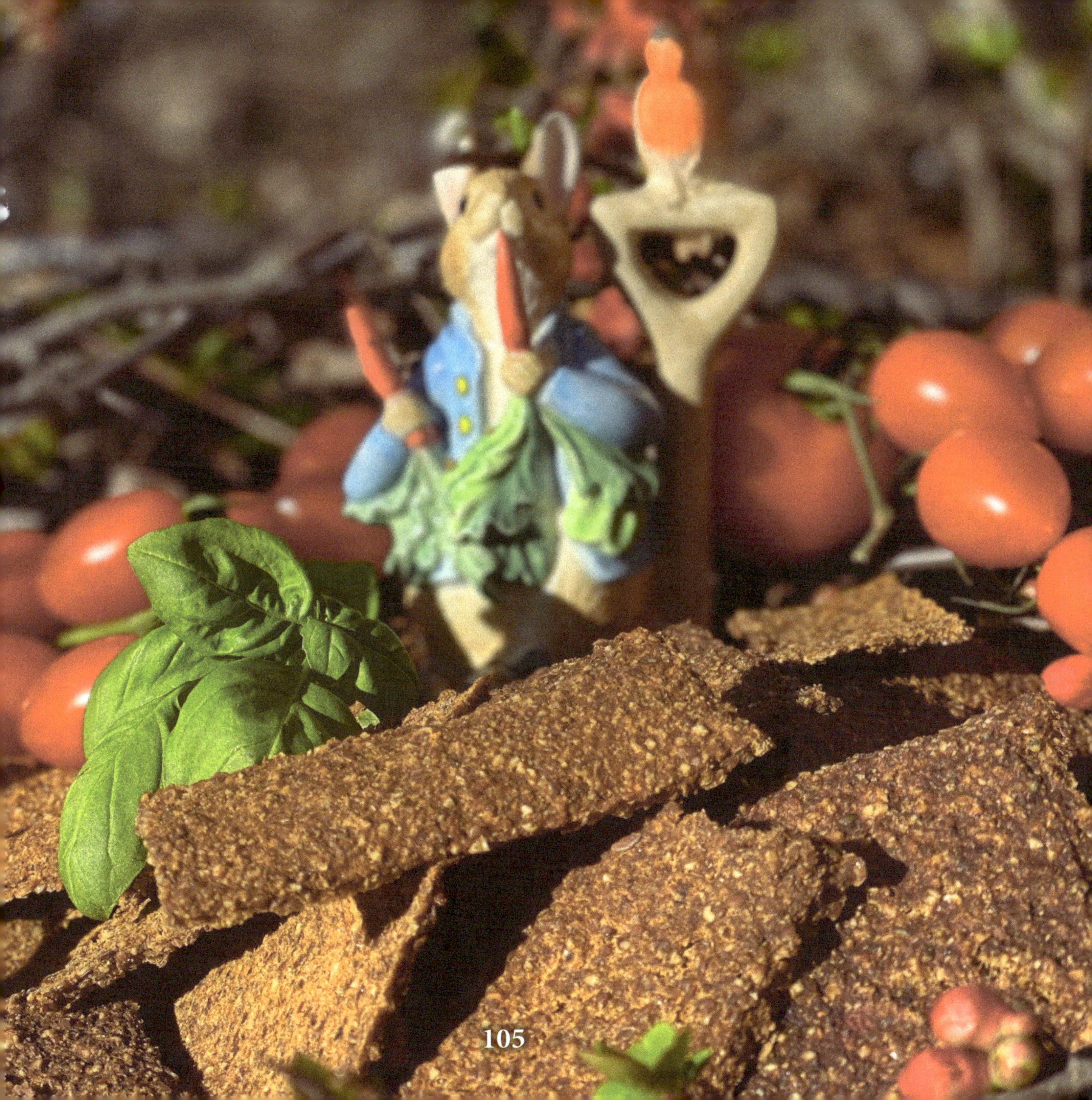

27

Fancy little PIZZA-like crackers

Many people's favorite savory treat… PIZZA!

Many kids love the thought of such a takeaway dinner, don't you agree? It may sound like a very special treat to them. Not all pizzas are created equal though. Most commercial pizzas are made with unhealthy ingredients, including the highly refined dough and heavily processed meat. Pizza also tends to be extremely high in calories.

I believe that just as with any other food it is about how you make it. It does not have to be all cheesy & salty & pepperoni sausage to taste great to kids. Let's ask your little ones which toppings they fancy. Let them help to decorate with cute cherry tomatoes, sliced/diced peppers and onions, mushrooms, olives cut into tiny rings, florets of broccoli and cauliflower, sweetcorn, or green peas… The basil and tomato flavored cracker base mix, mentioned on the previous page, invokes that Italian deliciousness of the all-round crowd-pleaser that pizza can be. Let's top it up with help from your kids and create a new raw healthy snack they will love.

Ingredients:

This recipe can be very simple or quite complex. You decide! Much may depend on what your fridge holds.

3-5 parsnips

Some tomatoes (or tomato purée)

1 level tablespoon of raw coconut oil

Mixed raw seeds – use sesame, sunflower, or flax seeds (brown flax above all others gives a 'bread' like feel to these crackers)

Pinch of sea salt

A handful of fresh basil leaves

Sprouts of grains or pulses would be on MY list of my basic ingredients too.

Optional extras for the pizza cracker mixture:

Garlic

Thyme / rosemary / oregano

Fresh sprouts such as buckwheat or lentils

Onions / scallions

Zucchini

Bell peppers of all colors

Celery stalks or pulp from leftover celery juicing

Carrots

Broccoli

Cauliflower

Aubergine

Sweet potato

Process

As you can see… one can hide many Vs for veg in a P for pizza. You can use as many or as few as you like. This creation of recipes has huge potential for versatility. Even fruits such as apples can be added to the blend. Our noble ambition is to promote ultimate health for your kids. Options for healthy toppings: Cherry tomatoes, peppers, onions, mushrooms, black or green olives, florets of broccoli, and cauliflower, sweetcorn or green peas.

For extra adventurous 'toppers': crushed cashews soaked in water, rinsed well, and finally coated with some yeast flakes can add a hint of a cheesy flavor to your little pizza. You can recreate the 'stringy cheese look' with shredded zucchini. To make the blended cracker mix: place all the ingredients in the blender with a cup of warm water and blend until almost smooth. Decide what size you want your little pizzas to be. I would suggest starting with one big heaped spoon of mixture for each little pizza. Place it in the palm of your hand, roll into a little ball, place on a silicone dehydrator sheet, and gently 'press' from above to create little pancake-like flat circles. Top them up with colorful raw toppings.

Place in the dehydrator. Dry at 113 degrees F (45 degrees C) for approx. 5 hours. Check upon your little pizzas, peel off the silicone sheets if possible. They will finish drying faster on a bare mesh. Dehydrate for 4-5 hours more. Check upon your creations again – if dehydrated to your liking, store them in an airtight box after a brief cooling down period. If they need drying for a little longer, you know what to do.

Thank crackers it's Friday!

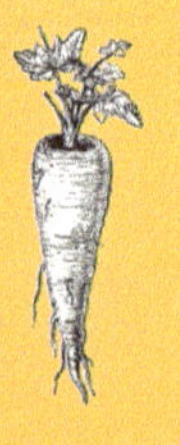
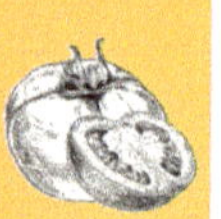
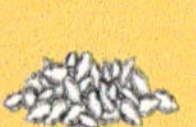
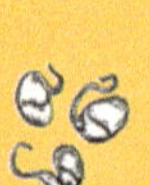

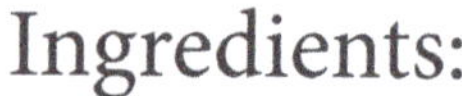

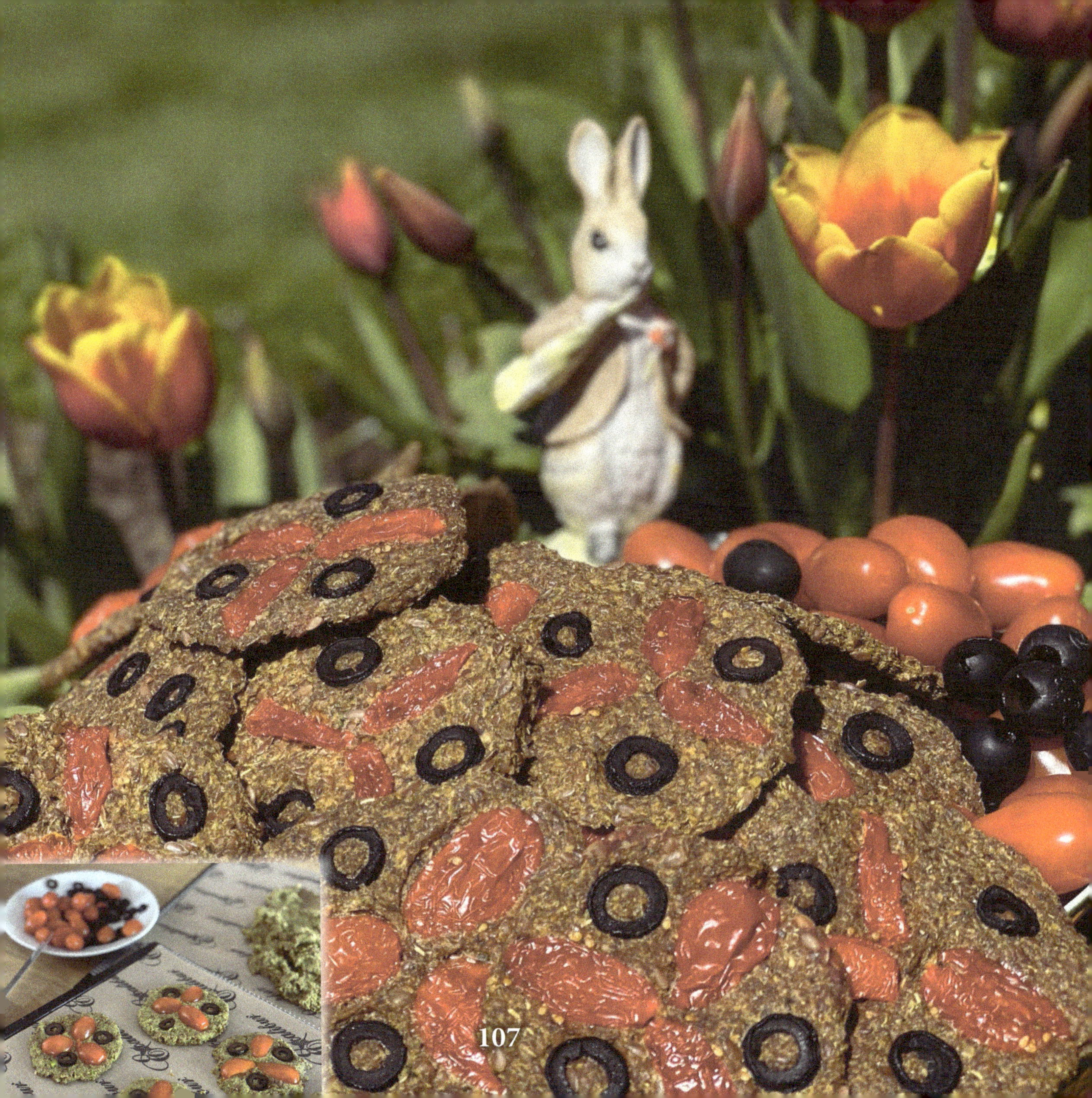

28

Flavorful CAULIFLOWER, CUMIN and RED BELL PEPPER

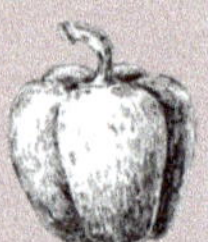

Feel like eating flowers?

This one from all the different 'flowers' I personally eat, is most likely the one your kids already know.

Cauliflower is loaded with vitamin C, which helps our bodies absorb iron—a critical nutrient in the growing bodies of kids. Cauliflower is also a great source of vitamin K and B vitamins and is rich in antioxidants. Got a constipated baby? Cauliflower might just help things, ahem, move along.

Cauliflower comes in a range of colors and varieties. Green cauliflower contains chlorophyll and more than twice as much vitamin C as the white variety; purple cauliflower is high in anthocyanins (an antioxidant), and orange cauliflower is high in beta-carotene, which aids eye, skin, and immune health.

Bell peppers (technically fruits not veggie) are so rich in vitamin A and C and have a wonderful flavor. Cumin seed supports healthy digestion and is a very iron-dense spice. This powerful seed has antibacterial and antioxidant properties. Cumin has been used traditionally in medicine for centuries. According to the Ayurveda, it is balancing for all three doshas.*

Ingredients:

1 medium to large cauliflower

2-3 red bell peppers

3 carrots

Pinch of sea salt

350 g of raw sunflower seeds (or a mix of yellow flaxseeds, sesame seeds with sunflower seeds)

Lemon juice (half a peeled lemon)

Optional:

Tahina

Apples

Black pepper

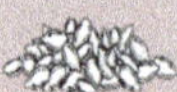

Process

Cut the cauliflower into smaller pieces and place it in a blender together with bell peppers, carrots, salt, seeds, lemon juice, and up to a cup of filtered water. Blend until you like the texture of the mixture.

Spread the blended cracker mix evenly on the Teflex sheet placed on the dehydrator tray. Once spread evenly (think thin pizza crust) try to score the mix with the side of the spatula or blunt knife into slices or squares. If the consistency is still too runny – dehydrate it for a couple more hours and score it once the cracker mix thickens (meaning it's drier). Dry at 113 degrees F (45 degrees C) for approx. 5 hours. Check your crackers, flip them and peel off the sheets if possible. Peeling the crackers off sheets and leaving them on a bare mesh of dehydrator tray makes drying much faster – hence I try to peel the cracker mix from the sheets as soon as it's possible. Dehydrate for 4-5 hours more. Recheck the crackers and, if crispy-dry, store them in airtight boxes after a brief cooling down. If drying for a little longer is needed, you know what to do.

Cracker time!

---

* Ayurvedic healing is an ancient Indian system based on a natural and holistic approach to physical and mental health. Within that system, doshas are energy patterns that flow around the body and determine who we are and how we feel.

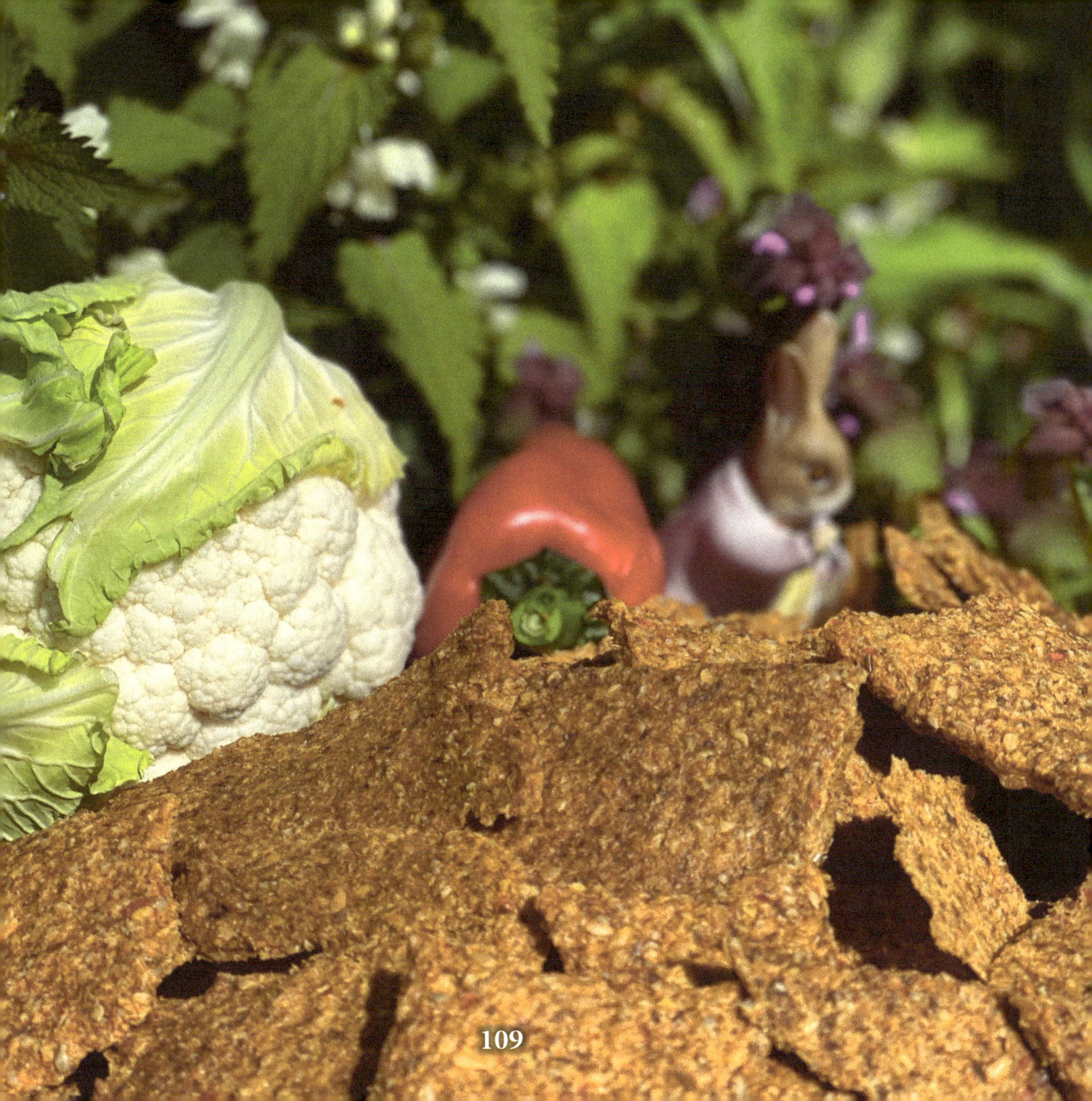

29

Enticing "cheesy" CHIVES with CASHEW

I have to warn you, these crackers are quite rich in taste, calories and… ok – I admit it – hard to stop eating.

I make them on special occasions or when having friends over, as they are a great party snack and go so well with many other items on party buffet menus. (As this book is mostly about crackers for children, I will not mention here that these go well with wine and cheese…anyway… that's the feedback so far! I would not know as I personally consume neither cheese nor alcohol.)

As with the crackers on the following six pages – one of the main ingredients is a sulfur-rich vegetable. Chives, when growing, look so innocent, almost like common grass, but they are delicious and healing. Did you ever try such a simple meal as buttered bread sprinkled with finely chopped chives? Well, that was what my mama gave me when I was a small girl running in the gardens, not willing to sit and eat. An easy on-the-go meal in those days. Chives grow fast and easily. Try to grow them in a pot on your balcony or windowsill. When they blossom, a beautiful purple flower appears-which is, by the way, edible too. So pretty as a garnish!

Ingredients:

500 g of raw cashew nuts

Half cup of yeast flakes (better start with less… you can increase the ratio of yeast in this recipe over time, once you know your kids can handle the flavor)

2 big handfuls of fresh chives (as an alternative to fresh chives one could use spring onions, although it is the second-best for me when it comes to flavor in this crackers)

3-5 parsnips

2 apples

1 medium lemon

Pinch of Himalaya salt

1 level tablespoon of raw coconut oil

Optional:

*Feel free to add some **broccoli and carrots***

Process

Soak the cashew nuts for 4-6 hours, and rinse thoroughly before using in this recipe… Peel the lemon, cut it in half and remove the seeds. Cut the parsnips into 3-5 cm bits before adding them to blender with the rest of the ingredients and half a cup of filtered water, adding more if needed.

Blend until you like the texture.

I personally like to see the little white bits of cashews in my crackers, so I add half of the total amount of nuts for this recipe into the blender only towards the very end of blending. As they are softened from soaking, they blend fast and easily anyway.

Spread the blended cracker mix evenly on the Teflex sheet placed on the dehydrator tray. Once spread evenly (think thin pizza crust) try to score the mix with the side of the spatula or blunt knife into slices or squares. If the consistency is still too runny – dehydrate it for a couple more hours and score it once the cracker mix thickens (meaning it's drier). Dry at 113 degrees F (45 degrees C) for approx. 5 hours. Check your crackers, flip them and peel off the sheets if possible. Peeling the crackers off sheets and leaving them on a bare mesh of dehydrator tray makes drying much faster – hence I try to peel the cracker mix from the sheets as soon as it's possible. Dehydrate for 4-5 hours more. Recheck the crackers and, if crispy-dry, store them in airtight boxes after a brief cooling down. If drying for a little longer is needed, you know what to do.

Chill and crack the cracker!

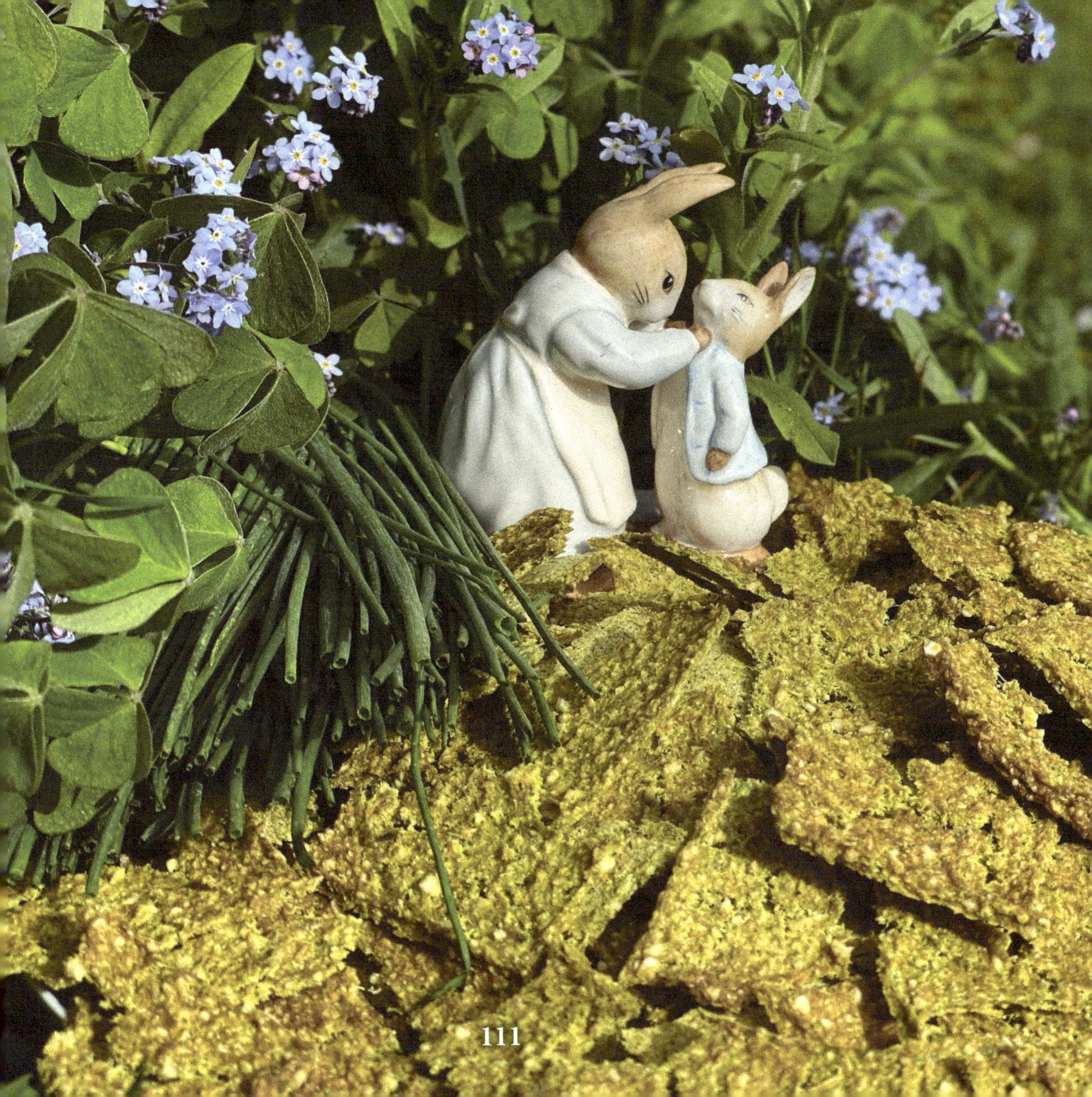

30

Funky LEEK and GREEN PEA

There is something about leeks…

In Ancient Rome, the leek was considered superior to onion and garlic.

It seems leek was the favorite vegetable of Emperor Nero: he consumed leek in his soup, or raw in oil, and believed leek was beneficial to the quality of his voice.

The leek is in the national emblem of Wales and plays an important role in a number of old legends about St.David, the patron saint of that country. At some point an image of the leek made it on the British £1 coin.

As I said, there is something about LEEKS!

There is no doubt that adding leek to your kid's plate is beneficial to health. The unique combination of flavonoids and sulfur-containing nutrients makes an allium vegetable such as a leek, a great choice for a base for a healthy savory snack or meal. The taste of green peas matched with the unique sweetness of leeks in these crackers makes them delicious. If you are not sure, just test this recipe.

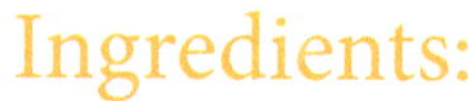

Ingredients:

5 big leeks

700 g of fresh green peas (if the worst comes to the worst — frozen is fine)

Pinch of Himalaya salt

1 level tablespoon of raw coconut oil

300 g of golden flaxseed

Optional:

1-2 parsnips
1-2 yellow or red apples
broccoli florets/ sprouts
radish sprouts

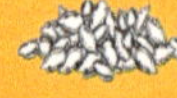

Process

The edible portion of the leek is the white base as well as the green parts. After washing, cut the leek into sections approx. 3 cm long before placing them in the blender. Add the rest of the ingredients together with a cup of warm filtered water and blend until you like the consistency of the cracker mix.

Spread the blended cracker mix evenly on the Teflex sheet placed on the dehydrator tray. Once spread evenly (think thin pizza crust) try to score the mix with the side of the spatula or blunt knife into slices or squares. If the consistency is still too runny – dehydrate it for a couple more hours and score it once the cracker mix thickens (meaning it's drier). Dry at 113 degrees F (45 degrees C) for approx. 5 hours. Check your crackers, flip them and peel off the sheets if possible. Peeling the crackers off sheets and leaving them on a bare mesh of dehydrator tray makes drying much faster – hence I try to peel the cracker mix from the sheets as soon as it's possible. Dehydrate for 4-5 hours more. Recheck the crackers and, if crispy-dry, store them in airtight boxes after a brief cooling down. If drying for a little longer is needed, you know what to do.

Keep calm and cracker!

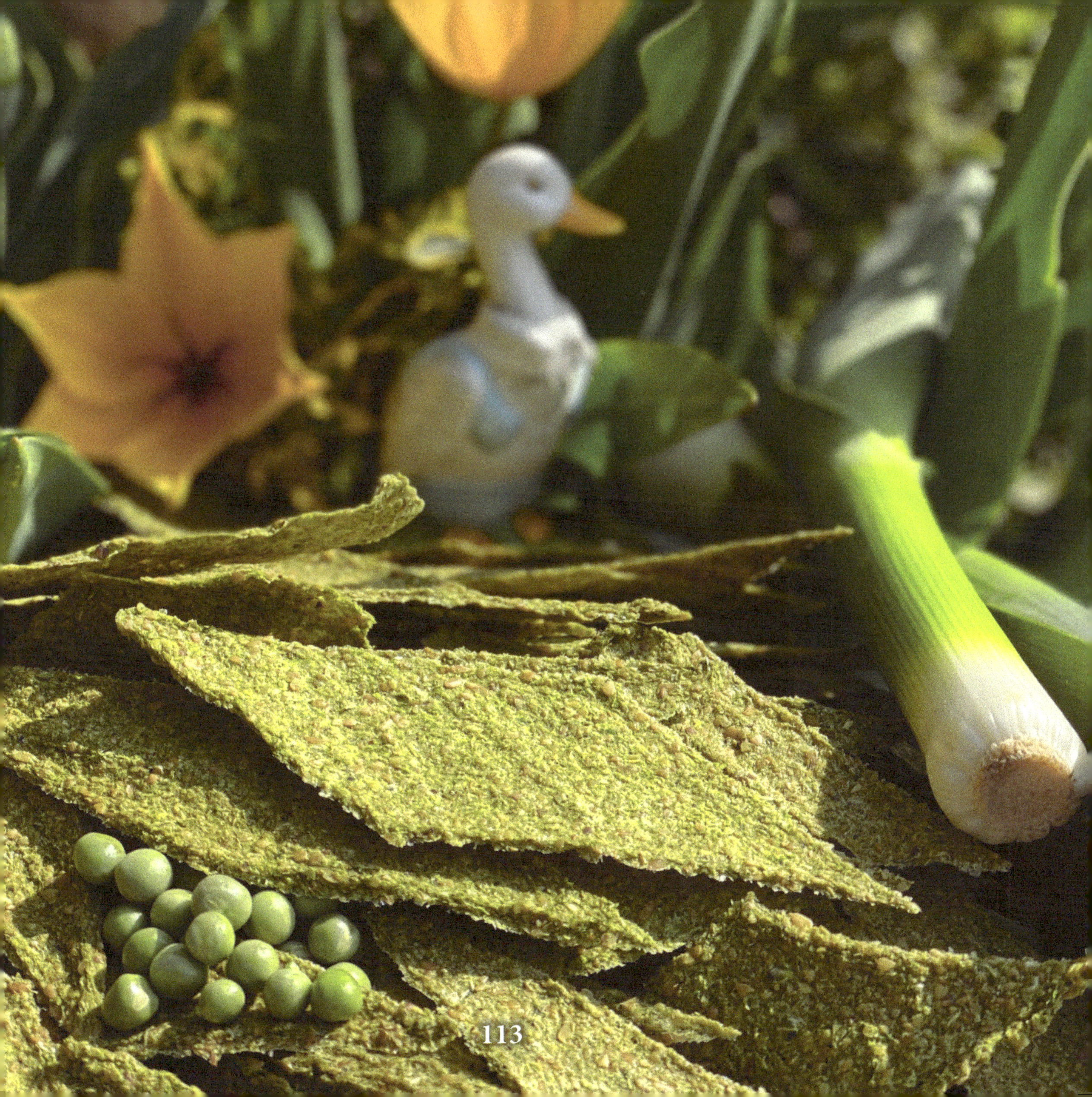

31

Charming RED ONION and CHIA seeds

It took me years in my youth to embrace raw onions on my plate. Now I will not let go. Love them all! Red, white, yellow, spring… Raw onions are a food for longevity and vibrant health. Close to zero calories and with a very long list of health benefits.

Onions belong to 'sulfur foods'- together with garlic, arugula, hot peppers, pine nuts, pine needles, aloe vera, watercress, radishes, etc. Our body needs sulfur. Sulfur aids the proper formation of proteins associated with connective tissues, hormones, enzymes, antibodies. It also contributes to healthy hair, nails, skin as well as helping to heal burns and scars. So yes, onions are yet another superfood.

Red onions are extra sweet and quite mild in taste compared to some other sulfur foods I have mentioned, so you may be surprised to find out that your kids like these red-onion-based crackers. (Tip: Perhaps try not to mention the "onion" word when you present these crackers for the first time.)

Let's call them simply "purple" crackers.

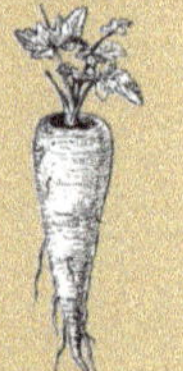

Ingredients:

5-7 big red onions

3-5 parsnips

3-5 red apples

1 -2 cups of chia seeds

1 level tablespoon of coconut oil

Pinch of Himalaya salt (or a big spoon of yeast flakes)

Optional:

A cup of raw sunflower seeds

Process

Place the parsnips, apples, coconut oil, and salt into a blender together with up to a cup of filtered water. Whizz the blender until the parsnip is chopped into smaller bits. Add halved red onions and all the seeds. Continue until you like the consistency and 'structure' of the blended cracker mix.

Spread the blended cracker mix evenly on the Teflex sheet placed on the dehydrator tray. Once spread evenly (think thin pizza crust) try to score the mix with the side of the spatula or blunt knife into slices or squares. If the consistency is still too runny – dehydrate it for a couple more hours and score it once the cracker mix thickens (meaning it's drier). Dry at 113 degrees F (45 degrees C) for approx. 5 hours. Check your crackers, flip them and peel off the sheets if possible. Peeling the crackers off sheets and leaving them on a bare mesh of dehydrator tray makes drying much faster – hence I try to peel the cracker mix from the sheets as soon as it's possible. Dehydrate for 4-5 hours more. Recheck the crackers and, if crispy-dry, store them in airtight boxes after a brief cooling down. If drying for a little longer is needed, you know what to do.

By the way… did you know that chia seeds are a great source of omega-3-fatty acids and fiber?

Love them in crackers as they add that extra bursting crispy sensation if dried properly.

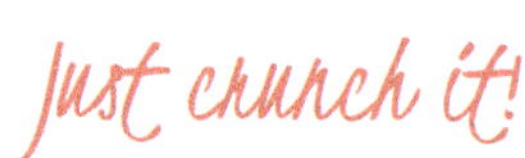

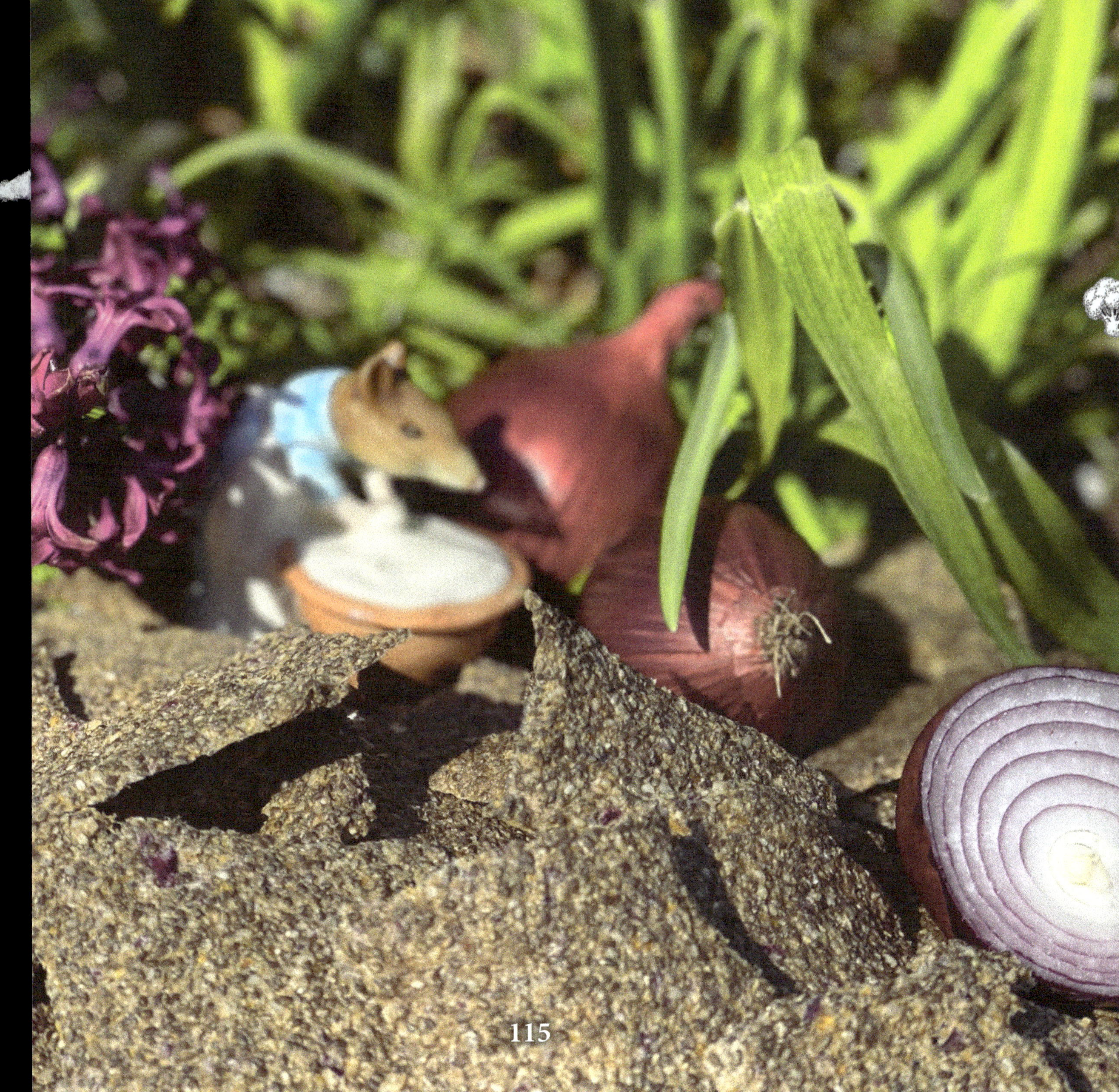

32

Gourmet BROCCOLI with sprouted MUNGO BEANS and GARLIC

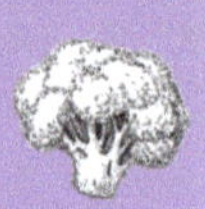

Do you feel your kids crave sugar? Are they often asking for sugary snacks or drinks? Broccoli can come to help! This wonderful dark green vegetable is rich in chromium, which helps to optimize insulin activity and hence help fight sugar addiction.

And yes, of course, vitamin C, vitamin A, calcium for stronger bones are just a few of the extra benefits I will name. Are you familiar with sprouting? If not – have a look at page 20 in this book for more whys and hows…

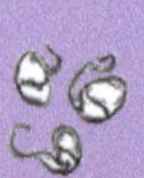

Mungo beans are very easy to sprout. These little beans are one of the best plant-based sources of protein. They're rich in essential amino acids such as phenylalanine, leucine, isoleucine, valine, lysine, and arginine. Essential amino acids are those that your body is unable to produce on its own.

The process of sprouting changes the nutritional composition of beans. Sprouted beans contain fewer calories and more free amino acids and antioxidants than unsprouted ones and are much easier to digest. I consider sprouts a superfood. They are full of antioxidants, minerals, and fiber too.

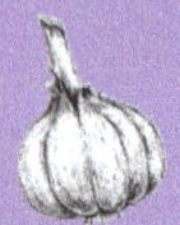

What's more, sprouting reduces levels of phytic acid, which is sometimes called an 'anti-nutrient.' Antinutrients can reduce the absorption of minerals like zinc, magnesium, and calcium.

In fact, feel free to replace the whole broccoli in this recipe with fresh broccoli sprouts (approx. 4 cups of sprouted broccoli seeds) for extra healing and 'magic' potential. (For a more detailed 'how' check my online blog post focused on broccoli seed sprouting.)

Ingredients:

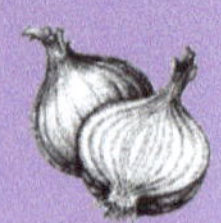

One whole fresh organic broccoli (stalks are fine to use too)

Cup of sprouted mungo beans

2-4 garlic cloves

1 big onion (red or white)

2-3 parsnips

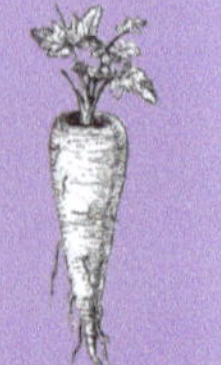

300 g of raw seeds of your choice

1 level tablespoon of raw coconut oil

Optional:

tomatoes/ tomato purée/ sundried tomatoes

A few celery stalks or pulp leftover from celery juicing.

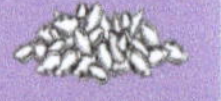

Process

Place all the ingredients in the blender together with up to a cup of filtered water.

Blend until you like the resulting texture.

Spread the blended cracker mix evenly on the Teflex sheet placed on the dehydrator tray. Once spread evenly (think thin pizza crust) try to score the mix with the side of the spatula or blunt knife into slices or squares. If the consistency is still too runny – dehydrate it for a couple more hours and score it once the cracker mix thickens (meaning it's drier). Dry at 113 degrees F (45 degrees C) for approx. 5 hours. Check your crackers, flip them and peel off the sheets if possible. Peeling the crackers off sheets and leaving them on a bare mesh of dehydrator tray makes drying much faster – hence I try to peel the cracker mix from the sheets as soon as it's possible. Dehydrate for 4-5 hours more. Recheck the crackers and, if crispy-dry, store them in airtight boxes after a brief cooling down. If drying for a little longer is needed, you know what to do.

To cracker or not to cracker?!

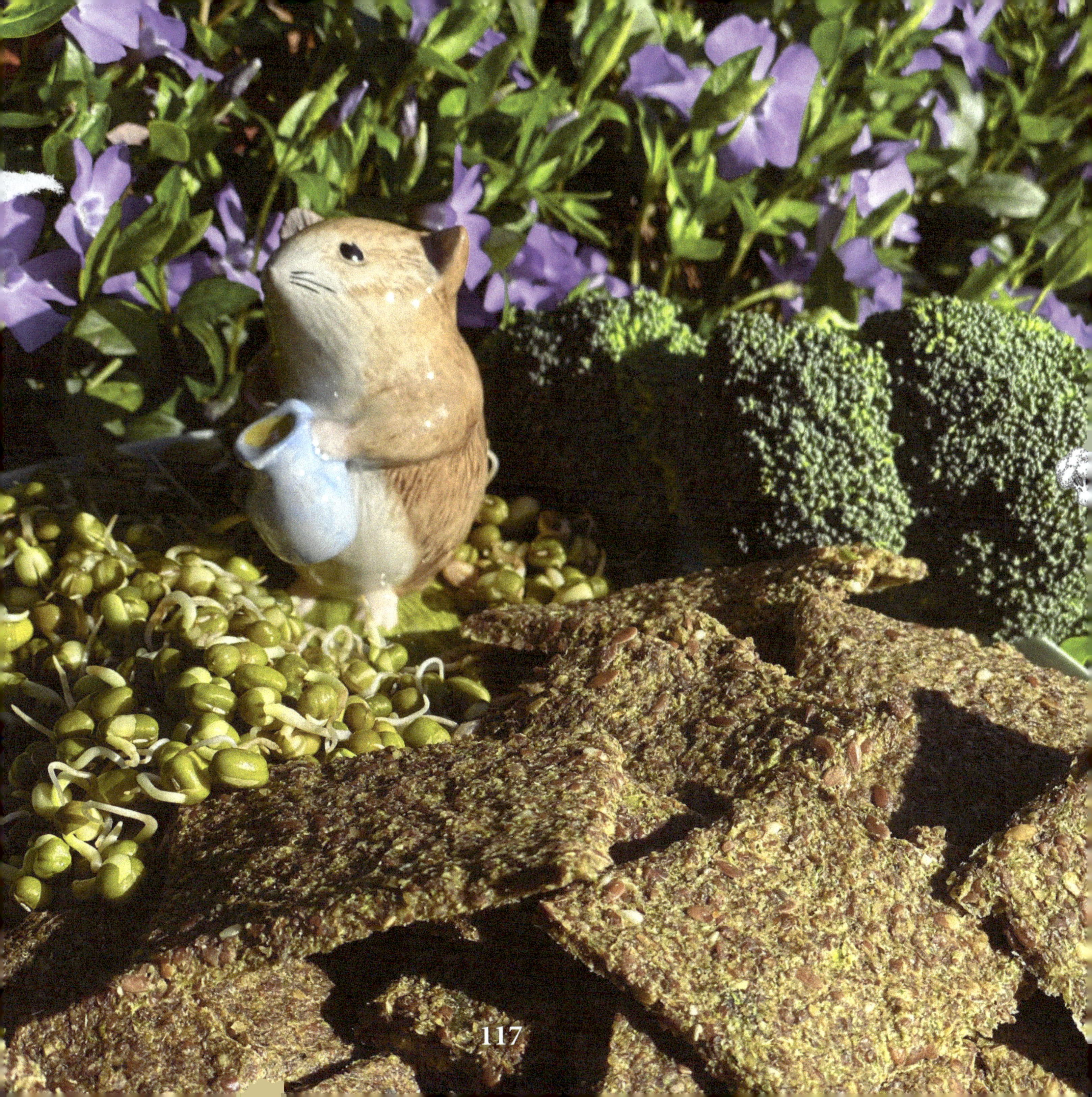

33

A "Delicate OLIVE meets The Cracker" adventure

Genesis 8:11 "The dove came to him toward evening, and behold, in her beak was a freshly picked olive leaf. So Noah knew that the water was abated from the earth…" There you have it… thousands of years ago the olive tree was around and recognized as very valuable. Looking at olive trees I find them to be absolutely beautiful. Each one of them is a unique masterpiece of Mother Nature, so very special. They grow slowly and are incredibly drought tolerant (if allowed to grow naturally, an olive tree may reach a height of 2 meters in 15 years.) Traditionally, the olive tree is a symbol of peace and friendship, an association which began in Ancient Greece…

Legend has it that Zeus proposed a contest between Athena and Poseidon for the control of Athens. Poseidon smashed his three-pronged trident upon the hard rock of the Acropolis, which unleashed spring, whilst Athena produced an olive tree, with its silvery-green leaves and abundance of rich fruits. The Athenians chose Athena's gift and in turn the olive tree has remained a much-loved part of Greek life ever since! I hope you like olives too. In case the answer is yes, try this wonderful olive-based delicate delicacy. You will need:

Ingredients:

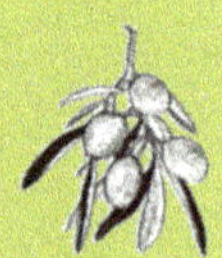

2-3 cups of olives (pitted, choose the ones you like)

A couple of broccoli florets

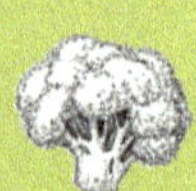

5-7 big celery stalks including their green leaves

2-4 parsnips

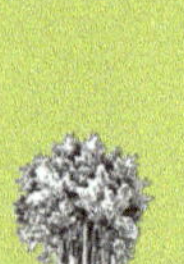

1 cup of sprouted buckwheat

Pinch of sea salt (optional, also depends on how salty your olives are)

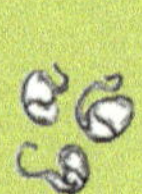

300 g of raw sunflower seeds, or mixed raw seeds

1 level tablespoon of raw coconut oil

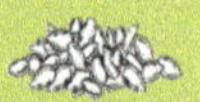

Process

Cut celery stalks into 3-4 cm sticks and place them in a blender together with the broccoli, parsnip, buckwheat sprouts, coconut oil, salt, a cup of water. Blend for two minutes, adding more water if necessary. Add olives and raw seeds and continue blending until the cracker mix is a nice texture, with little bits of olive still visible.

Spread the blended cracker mix evenly on the Teflex sheet placed on the dehydrator tray. Once spread evenly (think thin pizza crust) try to score the mix with the side of the spatula or blunt knife into slices or squares. If the consistency is still too runny – dehydrate it for a couple more hours and score it once the cracker mix thickens (meaning it's drier). Dry at 113 degrees F (45 degrees C) for approx. 5 hours. Check your crackers, flip them and peel off the sheets if possible. Peeling the crackers off sheets and leaving them on a bare mesh of dehydrator tray makes drying much faster – hence I try to peel the cracker mix from the sheets as soon as it's possible. Dehydrate for 4-5 hours more. Recheck the crackers and, if crispy-dry, store them in airtight boxes after a brief cooling down. If drying for a little longer is needed, you know what to do.

Olives are high in vitamin E and several antioxidants, which are good for heart health. They protect against osteoporosis and cancer, and help fight inflammation and infections caused by bacteria. They are a good source of monounsaturated fats and contain dietary fibers, vitamins B1, B3, B6, calcium, iron, and copper.

Unsalted olives can be added to the diets of kids and babies at the very beginning of the weaning journey, the nutritional benefits are many.

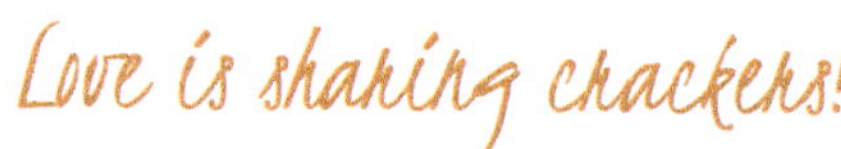
Love is sharing crackers!

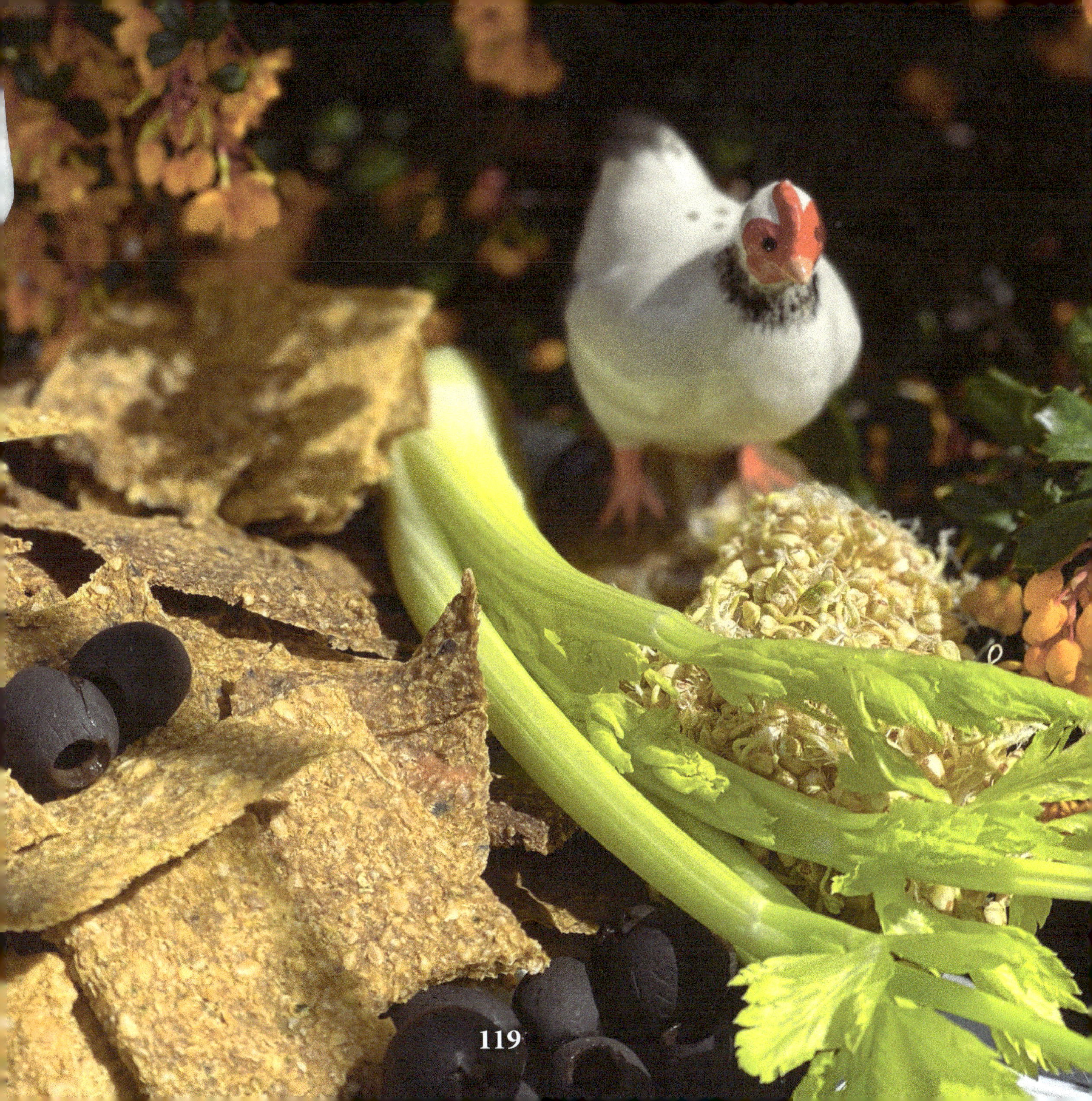

34

Bonus recipe:
Zesty LEMON and COCONUT

What do lemons mean to me? I think they are SUNSHINE on a tree.

Recently I received a beautiful surprise: someone who cares about me gifted me a LEMON TREE. It made me so happy, a perfect gift! For years now, I have consumed one lemon a day. Deep inside I know that's what my body wants. I can't wait to add safe untreated lemon peel to my crackers from my own lemon harvest.

We all know lemons are a great source of vitamin C. If you find yourself craving a lemon the chances are your body might be anemic. Lemons help the absorption of iron and calcium in the stomach, and in general aid digestion. They help to boost energy as well as immunity. Lemons are a wonderful antibacterial remedy for skin problems or a sore throat. To drink a glass of lemon water first thing in the morning is a valuable practice to try and apply long term. I often carry a lemon essential oil in my bag as the beautiful scent of lemon helps me relax and elevates my mood. Lemons are simply wonderful. I couldn't resist adding this bonus recipe inspired by them.

Ingredients:

6/7 medium parsnips

3-4 medium or 2-3 big lemons peeled deseeded

4 Golden Delicious apples

200 g of desiccated shredded coconut

1 level tablespoon of raw coconut oil

1 cup of yellow raisins

If you have a ripe banana you can add one to the mix.

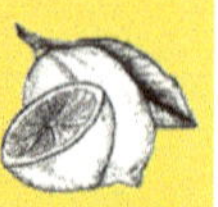

Variations to this recipe: I like to add a couple of pineapple cores to this coconut & lemon recipe, as the additional fiber makes the crackers even more crispy once dried fully.

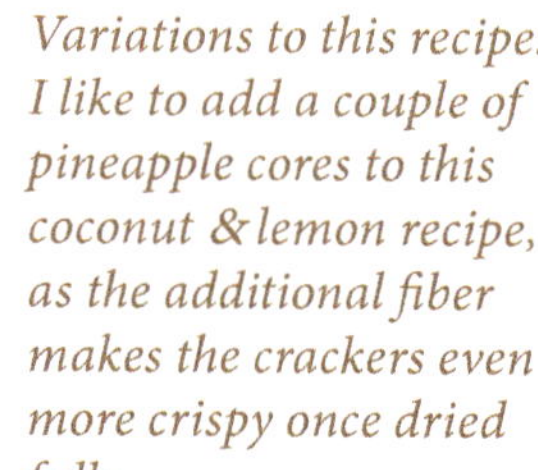

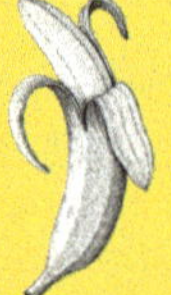

Process

Place the parsnips, apples, coconut oil, and a cup of filtered water into the blender. Blend until the hard ingredients are cut into small bits. Peel the lemons, cut into halves, and remove their seeds (as they would taste bitter in crackers). Add the lemon halves, desiccated coconut, and golden raisins to the blender. If you get a chance, soak the raisins for couple of hours and rinse them well before adding. Blend the cracker mix with the help of the blender's tamper until you like the texture of it.

Spread the blended cracker mix evenly on the Teflex sheet placed on the dehydrator tray. Once spread evenly (think thin pizza crust) try to score the mix with the side of the spatula or blunt knife into slices or squares. If the consistency is still too runny – dehydrate it for a couple more hours and score it once the cracker mix thickens (meaning it's drier). Dry at 113 degrees F (45 degrees C) for approx. 5 hours. Check your crackers, flip them and peel off the sheets if possible. Peeling the crackers off sheets and leaving them on a bare mesh of dehydrator tray makes drying much faster – hence I try to peel the cracker mix from the sheets as soon as it's possible. Dehydrate for 4-5 hours more. Recheck the crackers and, if crispy-dry, store them in airtight boxes after a brief cooling down. If drying for a little longer is needed, you know what to do.

You really can't go wrong by adding a ripe banana to the blend. Try to add a cup of (soaked and well rinsed) cashew nuts to make this recipe more calorie dense. Cashew nuts add that creamy undertone and 'almost like cheesecake' luxurious feel. For fancy optional adds-on consider true vanilla essence/pods and maybe dates.

Let's cracker dance!

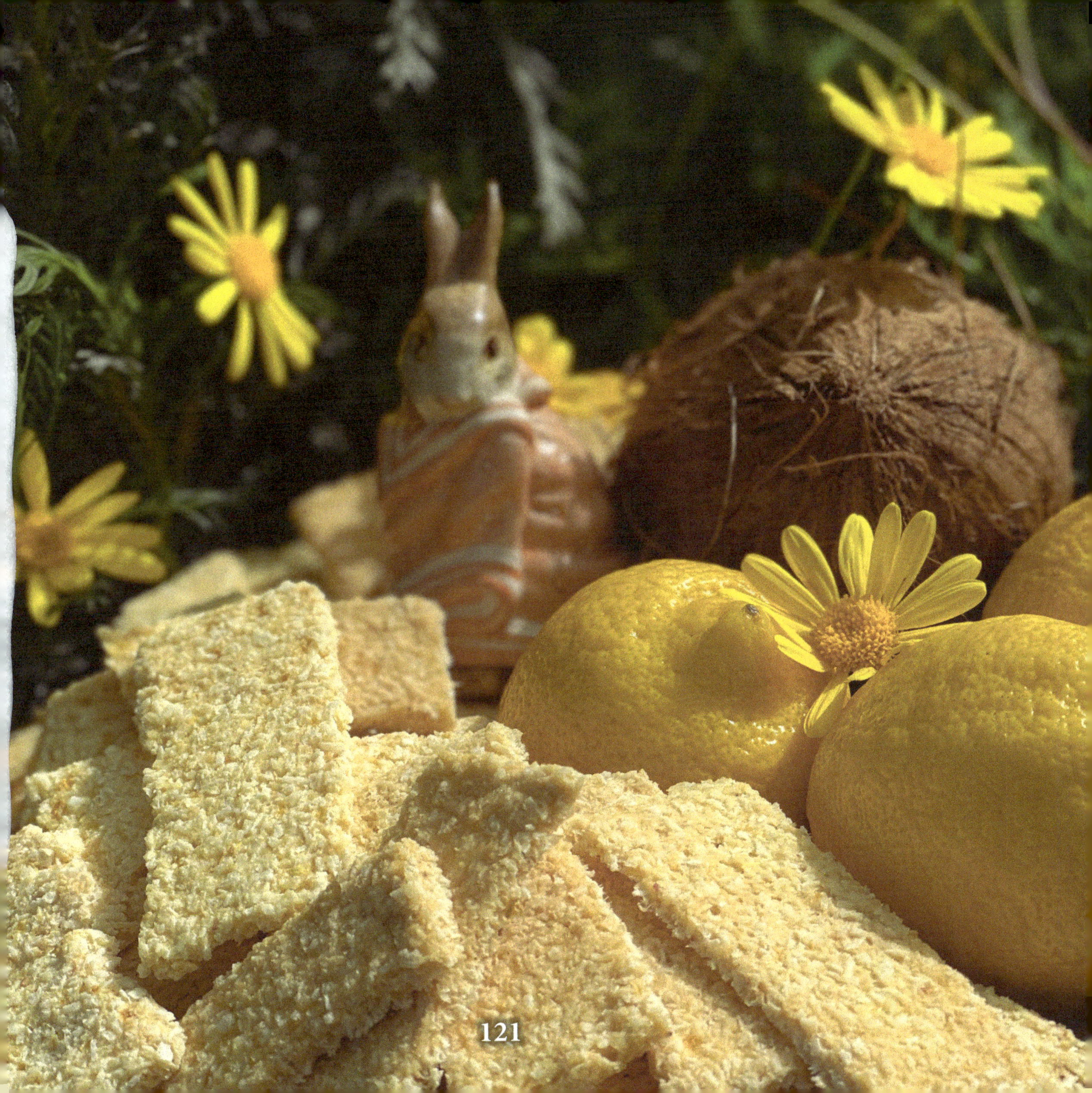

Be Yourself.

...this is possibly the most UN-EXACT and UN-COOK COOKBOOK you have ever seen.

What?? How Cheeky of Margo… right?

What I mean is – I am quite certain one does not have to follow to the T the amounts of the ingredients I mentioned in each recipe to make a great cracker. Trust me… I will not feel hurt if you do not fully follow everything I've written. In fact, feel free to modify ("fiddle with") each recipe and very likely the final product will still be a magnificent cracker. And it will be UNIQUE to YOU!

I think that's where the magic lies.

Feeling inspired and not worrying too much about doing it "right" makes you want to do it more… To come to this book again and again and keep 'crackering' to yours and your children's hearts' content.

And of course, 'un-cook' accords with the simple fact that we do not need to heat the ingredients to temperatures over 45 °C to make these crackers. The healthy, pure, natural ingredients are only being "dried" in conditions that preserve loads of nutrients in their original form. Hence we dare to call our crackers "raw."

PS: I should say, for those who skipped the general chapter about what my mad crackers are made of, that they consist of raw fruit, raw vegetables, raw seeds/nuts or sprouted seeds. As long as you stick to these (and abstain from sausages, bacon, M&Ms, cheese, chicken wings, or other crazy ingredients my husband would most likely think of/dream of throwing in and adding) – the above statement applies.

So yes, my cracker recipes are forgiving. A little less or a little more of something doesn't really matter. If you use ripe and clean ingredients, the outcome of goodness is guaranteed.

Please also get comfortable with substitutions. When ingredients in my recipe are not available to you try to replace them with something similar that is in season and ripe.

Make your 'own' extra yummy crackers: Example from Margo's Mad about Crackers Cracking Diary:

What a lovely morning. Woke up and felt thirsty for a biiiiig glass of fresh carrot juice. After practicing some brief gratitude I took seven carrots and juiced them directly into Nutribullet's jug, so as not to create extra dirty dishes. To make my fresh carrot juice even better I threw in a chunk of ginger, a slice of fresh pineapple, half a peeled lemon, and some ice cubes and whizzed using Nutribullet blender until smooth. Drank and enjoyed this divine refreshing drink slowly while planning what this new day will be about...

But, before the day really begins, this carrot pulp will not go to waste!

Decided not to freeze the pulp this time but went ahead and crafted orange flavor crackers for my sweet family. For this impromptu recipe, I used five parsnips, one peeled lemon, five peeled oranges (removed seeds from all the citruses), a level tablespoon of raw coconut oil, and one cup of raw chia seeds. Placed all into my Vitamix blender together with two pineapple cores from pineapples we had for dinner the other day. Added some filtered water and blended all the ingredients into a cracker mixture with a slight grainy texture. Once done blending, I spread some of the cracker mix over 2 Teflex Excalibur

***

How It All Started... and Healthy Snacks.

After my first book GO WILD, I didn't think an 'inner calling' and inspiration for the second one would happen so soon.

It started with a CRACKER...

I realized how much I enjoy nibbling on my own creations.

The feedback from people around me who tasted them was really positive and encouraging.

The flood of followers and fans started to grow.

I noticed my own passion was being raised to a new level.

After spending some time with a beautiful family with three kids under the age of six and making crackers for them almost on daily basis (that was my chance to test the new combos and ideas), I realized how helpful and inspiring my ideas could potentially be to parents out there.

I became MAD about crackers...

I guess in the 'real world' it is not easy to find healthy snacks for kids that tick all the boxes.

Healthy...

Affordable...

Liked...

Easy to make and store...

Having a long shelf life (even though it seemed the big full box never lasted long enough).

Not too messy to eat or carry around...

Do people in your household tend to eat between meals, snacks that are at best non-nutritious and maybe even harmful?

This can make it easier for them to switch to the right ones... let the CRACKERING begin!

And yes, I wholeheartedly agree, fresh is the best. In my home and in places/households I get to work in, I aim to have a bowl of fruits on display, in a visible place, for kids to easily reach.

It makes my heart sing to see toddlers and kids enjoying eating fresh fruits and vegetables, asking for more, eating these life-giving gifts of nature, developing healthy eating habits, effortlessly making these food choices, setting their relationship with food to success mode for years to come.

Healthy kids move so much, burn calories AND grow at the same time. Foods – building blocks for their bodies – are super important. Each and every bite counts. Every meal/snack will either help them to grow and develop to their best potential or in the case of processed foods hinder that development (even though it's not something visible to our eyes, it is happening regardless.)

As an alternative to fresh fruit and vegetables I think crackers are the best! They have the potential to be LOVED BY YOUR KIDS... Especially those who are not great fans of fresh fruits and veggies.

They will never know they are actually eating raw vegetables when tasting these crackers!

Your quest to find the holy grail of healthy snacks for your entire family has led you to these recipes.

I have little confession to make. There is a part of me with the tendencies of a perfectionist… when I was looking at the images I created months ago for this book - that little critical voice in my mind that I tried to silence – kept whispering that I could still do better: intentionally blend the cracker "goo" a little less or a little more to make the crackers on the photographs look more appetizing… or wait for a better, sunnier day for the photo shoot… or for a different flower to bloom… My "today-self" with hundreds of trays of crackers 'under my belt', feels a long way away from where I was when I started, when I wasn't *completely happy.*

Then I took a deep breath... Many photographs which were in front of me (tons by the way – trying to choose one for each recipe wasn't the easiest task) brought back beautiful memories of my walks in an English springtime with nature waking up everywhere around me. And in a moment it struck me — my personal journey of making crackers has been and still is exciting, interesting and joy-bringing. I came a long way. It is and always will be a journey. There is no final destination. I know I will stick with it. My pictures will keep getting better. My crackers will get more photogenic if I want them to. And best of all… because of social media, I can share them with the world and those who are interested in joining in. One thing I can promise you: the crackers were and are still very yummy. Let's not judge the book by its cover and sometimes the cracker by the way it looks. It is what's inside that matters. And the crackers I made back then or/and this week are all made from ripe clean fruits and vegetables, they have threads of sun, wind, and earth in them, blended with the love I make each one of them with. It doesn't get better than that. I couldn't ask for more. I have found something I enjoy doing and sharing. Well, I LOVE to nibble on my own creations. And I sincerely hope you will too.

ACKNOWLEDGEMENTS

I have so many wonderful people (plants and babies too) to THANK for their support, motivation, and feedback on my creative journey. I would like to express my gratitude to all the little angels who were entrusted to my care. They are my sweet magical teachers and source of inspiration! Love and thanks to their parents — I am so grateful for your friendship and trust! Thank you dearest Julian and Zuzana for your LOVE, care, and most generous support on every step of the crackering journey. Jul you make me smile time and time again when you state, "I think these are my absolute favorite!" to each new batch I present to you.

Special thanks to Jacqueline, amazing editor, so talented, and (luckily for me) patient with my endless list of new ideas and amendments. Thank you dear Jean, Vicky, Cindy, Kia, Pali, Mirka for being such great cracker tasters! Your help with pictures too is invaluable.

Above all: THANK YOU beautiful Lara, Lyon, Ben, Wilf, Sophie, Saoirse, John, Cormac, Donnacha, Hassiba, Kenton and Atlas for being the kindest, most loving and supportive friends… despite the fact that sometimes all I want to talk about are BABIES, CRACKERS, and manifesting!

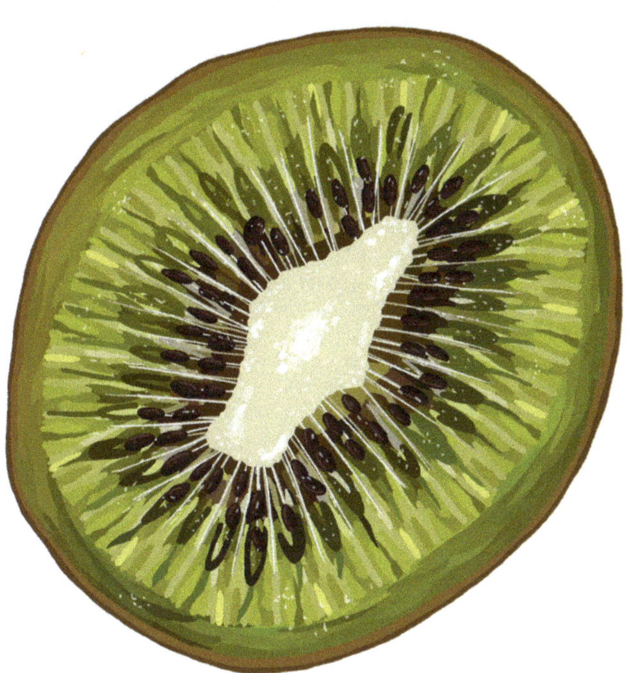

While sitting in your favorite chair and enjoying your own *Master-Cracker*, please post a review about your crackering and cracker eating experience. It will have a real impact on the life of this book and its humble author, and more people will get to read this, and cracker, thanks to you...

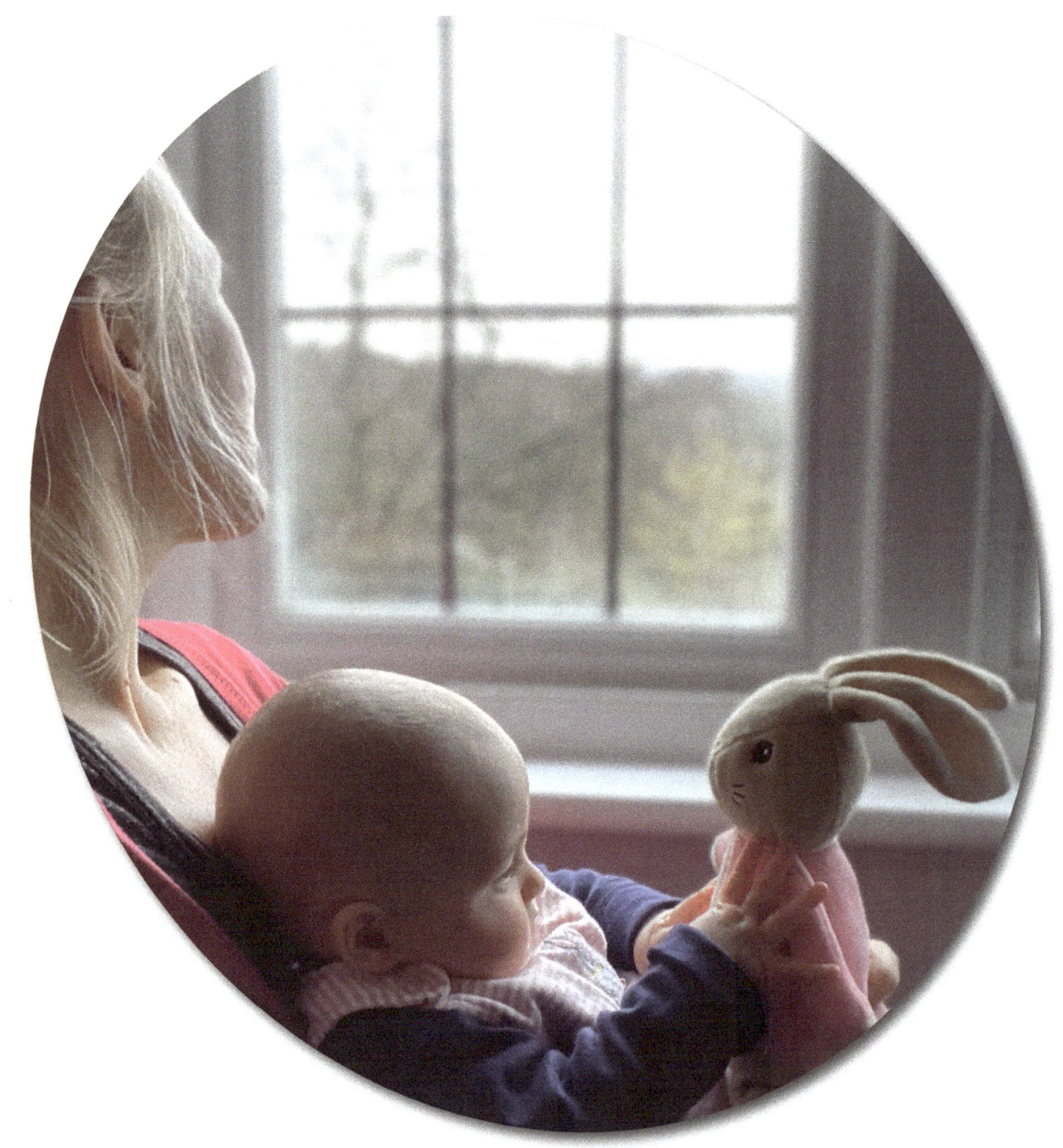

"LET'S MAKE CRACKERS NOT WAR!" Kenton Oxley